SAFETY

*principles, instruction,
and readings*

SAFETY

principles, instruction, and readings

ALTON L. THYGERSON
Brigham Young University

prentice-hall, inc., englewood cliffs, new jersey

© 1972 by Prentice-Hall, Inc., Englewood Cliffs, New Jersey

ISBN: P 0–13–785709–8
     C 0–13–785717–9

Library of Congress Catalog Card No.: 75–158196

10 9 8 7 6 5 4 3 2 1

Printed in the United States of America

prentice-hall, international, inc., london
prentice-hall of australia pty. ltd., sydney
prentice-hall of canada ltd., toronto
prentice-hall of india private ltd., new delhi
prentice-hall of japan, inc., tokyo

Dedicated to all the Thygersons

contents

preface

My goal in writing this book is to present a systematic account of the foundations of safety so that it is both understandable and interesting to readers with little previous knowledge of the subject; this goal has largely dictated the contents of the book. I'm certain there will not be perfect agreement among safety authorities concerning which topics should and should not have been chosen for extended treatment.

In comparison with other available textbooks the book devotes an unusual amount of space to defining the term "accident," exploring the concept of risk, analyzing accident proneness and scare techniques, presenting a framework for developing countermeasures of accident causal factors centered upon epidemiology and etiology, and giving a rationale for safety instruction. However, the book omits traditional content material of safe practices (home, school, work, etc.) which appears in other textbooks. Also absent are lists of safety rules; a book based on specific rules would be of encyclopedic size and such listings are generally incomplete.

Selected readings have been added to offer the reader exposure to the contributions of safety authorities. Such a compilation of readings also eases the difficulty of searching for excellent articles which are sometimes unavailable.

I am indebted to numerous persons. In some cases it has been possible to document this fact in specific citations and acknowledgements. In others no specific identification can be given.

The helpful cooperation of numerous publishers in giving permission to quote and to reprint is gratefully acknowledged. Specific permissions for which the author is most grateful are indicated in appropriate footnotes.

A remark by Samuel Johnson impresses me with its truth: that the best way to learn about a subject is to write a book.

SAFETY
principles, instruction, and readings

1 _why study about accidents?_

After reading this chapter, you should be able to:

1. _Define the term "accident," emphasizing preventability rather than chance._
2. _Point out reasons for studying about accidents._

Definition of an Accident

It is doubtful that any single definition would cover events called accidents. One definition reads, "An accident is an unplanned event frequently leading to undesirable effects, and is preceded by a preventable act(s) and/or unsafe condition(s)." According to this definition, accidents: (1) are unplanned, (2) lead frequently to undesirable effects, (3) are preventable, and (4) occur as a result of unsafe act(s) and/or unsafe condition(s). Let us examine these elements in detail.

AN UNPLANNED EVENT

The definition of the word "accident" hinders accident prevention efforts. For instance, medical science has long emphasized the resultant damage of a disease rather than its "unexpectedness"; this emphasis has proved rather successful. To many, the word "accident" implies that something unexpected and unpleasant occurred and that: it could not be helped, but was an accident; it was inevitable and could have happened to anyone;

_1_

it was unforeseen and thus uncontrollable; and it was not our responsibility and we are therefore not to be blamed. This definition of an accident as an "unplanned" or "unpredictable" occurrence implies an event which may be uncontrollable.

UNDESIRABLE EFFECTS

Tobacco smoking was not a recognized problem as long as most people smoked. Only when a large number of people decided that tobacco smoking was harmful (after considering the evidence) and said "Isn't it awful!" did smoking become a recognized problem. Awareness of a problem requires that we make a *value judgment,* a decision that the condition is "good" or "bad." A person's value judgment may define a condition as either undesirable, and therefore requiring change, or proper and acceptable. Consequently, what is called "undesirable" may vary from individual to individual, from situation to situation, even from culture to culture.

People in our society decide that accidents are unacceptable because they cause undesirable effects such as death, injury, and property damage. It should be noted that the ingestion of a polio virus or *bacillus botulinus* is not usually classified as an accident, whereas swallowing lye or an insecticide is. Such an inconsistency sets a definite limitation upon the definition of an accident. Undesirable or harmful effects are no longer the focal point in accident studies, but now have minor significance in the investigation of accident causation.

Death, injury, or property damage—consequences of an unplanned event—do not in themselves constitute the accident, but are the results. The consequences are merely the last in a series of happenings, each of which contributes something to the accident. For example, if a driver falls asleep at the wheel but awakes in time to avoid a collision, the event is not recorded as an accident. A study of these near accidents, however, could furnish clues to accident causation. The events recorded as accidents—those involving death, injury, or property damage—represent a very small percentage of the total consequences of unplanned happenings. Additional undesirable effects include anger, fear, and embarrassment, which are often correlated with both accidents and near accidents.

PREVENTABLE EVENTS

Until recently, everybody talked about the weather but nobody did anything about it. For instance, floods were simply a misfortune to be endured before the development of flood control. Now that we can exercise some control over the weather through new developments such as cloud-seeding and proper placement of dams, we see that a previously undesirable condition can be prevented. Similarly, an accident becomes a problem when we believe it can be avoided. Often the prevention of an accident can only be determined by trial-and-error. In the meantime, the accomplishments of accident prevention to date encourage us to try to avert the large death, injury, and property losses which result from accidents.

We note a significant trend toward emphasis on prevention of further loss after the event rather than on prevention of the accident. In the past, efforts to reduce accident losses have been made through the use of means such as education, prohibitions, and licensing which exert influence upon accident prevention. Today, several authorities believe that more emphasis should be placed upon those safeguards such as safety belts, steel-toed shoes, first aid, transportation of injured and other after-the-accident countermeasures.

UNSAFE ACT(S) AND/OR UNSAFE CONDITION(S)

A realistic appraisal of recent accident data clearly shows that *few* events labeled accidents really are accidents in that they are purely chance events.

Like other events, accidents are caused, and therefore, can be controlled when their causes are identified and understood. Frequently, accidents are not unforeseeable because most of them are not chance occurrences but rather reflect inefficiencies in the system. Accidents occur because people make mistakes. The statement that "80 percent of accidents are *caused* by human beings" may be simplistic and require confirming research. Human error frequently underlies unsafe conditions such as poor design, construction, and maintenance; therefore, most accidents are still attributable to human error.

Finally, it should be mentioned that several authorities suggest that the term "accident" be discarded. They believe it more reasonable to classify the resultant injuries as electrical, chemical, mechanical, etc. The misconceptions which accompany the term "accident" can also be avoided by this classification. In science if the cause of an event is known, that event is not an accident; most accident causes are known, but we still persist in calling them accidents. However, the use of the term may be too entrenched in the language for it to disappear.

John J. Brownfain makes a discerning observation about defining accidents:

> If we label all of life's unpleasant surprises as accidents, then we come to perceive ourselves as the playthings of fate and we cultivate a philosophy of carelessness and irresponsibility. On the other hand, if we look for causes and hold ourselves accountable for the mishaps in our lives, we become

people of resource and confidence, increasingly able to control the direction of events. If these conclusions are as true as I think they are, it matters very much how we define the word accident.[1]

Reasons for Studying About Accidents

AWARENESS

First, students should be aware of the main accident problems. Have you ever visited a place and then been surprised at how often you heard or read about that place afterwards? The place had been mentioned just as frequently before you visited it, but you never noticed these comments until you were acquainted with it; therefore, you found meaning in each reference because it related to something which had become familiar. Similarly, if we are aware of a particular accident problem we would notice each reference to it in the newspaper, possibly take time to read a magazine article about it, or become more attentive when it comes up in conversation. In this way we constantly increase our knowledge of a problem and the validity of our judgments about it.

FACTUAL KNOWLEDGE

All intelligent analysis must rest upon facts. It makes little sense to "discuss" an accident problem unless someone in the group knows what he is talking about. Although fact-gathering will not solve any problem automatically, it is impossible to analyze a problem until the facts have been collected, organized, and interpreted.

Misconceptions about safety and accidents exist because all the facts may not be known or presented. Unfortunately, these misconceptions and myths persist yet, in spite of educational efforts. (See Figures 1–1 and 1–2.) As a self-check for misconceptions, see how well you perform on the test in Table 1–1 on page 6.

UNDERSTANDING THE SCIENCE OF
ACCIDENT PREVENTION

It is valuable that we have a *general understanding of how and why accidents occur, how people are affected by accidents, and how we can deal with them.* These general understandings provide a frame of refer-

[1] John J. Brownfain, "When Is an Accident Not an Accident?" *Journal of the American Society of Safety Engineers* (September 1962), p. 20.

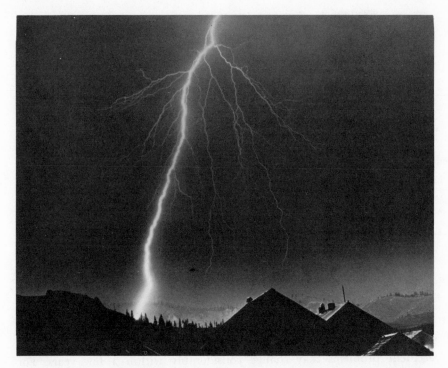

FIGURE 1–1 *Does lightning ever strike twice in the same place? Reproduced courtesy of the National Oceanic and Atmospheric Administration.*

ence within which we can catalog data and study specific problems. If one has a thorough understanding of the science of accident prevention, one can organize and analyze intelligently data on any particular accident. In addition, these general understandings help us interpret new data correctly and keep us up to date. Accident data often become obsolete and

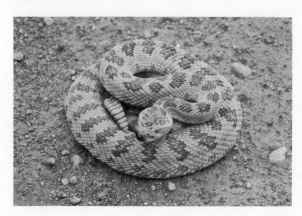

FIGURE 1–2 *Myths exist about the rattlesnake. The venom of bees, wasps, and hornets causes more deaths in the United States each year than are caused by the venom from the bite of a rattlesnake. Reproduced courtesy of the Utah Division of Fish and Game.*

TABLE 1–1   *Test on Safety Myths*

Which of the statements below are misconceptions in safety?

_____ 1. *Lightning never strikes twice in the same place.*
_____ 2. *Red is the hunter's best clothing color.*
_____ 3. *A silver spoon or silver coin will turn black after coming in contact with a poisonous mushroom.*
_____ 4. *Boiling or soaking poisonous mushrooms in salt water makes them safe.*
_____ 5. *A rattlesnake gives warning before striking.*
_____ 6. *The first procedure in saving a drowning person is to jump in the water.*
_____ 7. *It is impossible to stay afloat in water for long with clothes on.*
_____ 8. *If a boat overturns, you should swim to shore.*
_____ 9. *A drowning person always comes up for air three times.*
_____10. *Applying a tourniquet is the best way to stop bleeding.*
_____11. *Put butter on a burn.*
_____12. *Put beefsteak on a black eye or wound.*
_____13. *Put a cold knife on a bump on the head.*
_____14. *Blow smoke in the ear of a person with an earache.*
_____15. *Rub snow on frostbite.*
_____16. *The primary danger from leaking gas is asphyxiation.*
_____17. *Coffee will help sober up a drunk.*
_____18. *Smaller vehicles can stop in less time and distance than larger ones.*
_____19. *Pumping the brakes helps stop a car more quickly on dry pavement.*

Now turn to the article by Joyce de Cicco on pp. 82–87 for correct answers and explanations.

accident problems may change considerably within a few years. For example, there is change in concern about motorcycle and snowmobile death and injury statistics and a decrease in concern about abandoned refrigerators and ultra-thin plastic clothing covers as potential hazards. Yet, if the student understands the science of accident prevention, he will not find it hard to interpret new data and understand new accident trends.

Our attitudes and values determine the meanings we find in the facts we observe. A study of some widespread fallacious attitudes toward accidents may help show why people react to facts so differently and such a study may also help show why we may always have accident problems.

Listed are fallacious beliefs authored by Hein, Farnsworth, and Richardson:

1. The "other fellow" concept, whereby it is assumed that accidents happen to other people but won't happen to you.
2. The "your number's up" concept, whereby it is assumed that "when your number is up," you will get hurt and there is nothing you can do about it.
3. The "law of averages" concept, whereby accidents and injuries are shrugged off as due to inevitable statistical laws.
4. The "price of progress" concept, whereby accidents are rationalized as the inevitable price of scientific advancement.

5. The "spirit of '76" concept, whereby living dangerously is glorified and safety measures are regarded as "sissy."
6. The "act of God" concept, whereby accidents are seen as divinely caused —for punishment or for some purpose unknown to us.[2]

A SENSE OF PERSPECTIVE

Some people find the study of accidents upsetting. Just as people are frightened by all the diseases they find listed in a medical textbook, some students are disturbed by the great amount of expressed or implied criticism of our society that they find in a safety course. For others, awareness of imperfections which result in accidents may become an obsession. They are so distressed with the tragedy, suffering, and waste caused by an accident-plagued society that they fail to see more encouraging aspects of the total picture. We need a sense of perspective if we are to see without exaggeration or distortion.

APPRECIATION OF THE PROPER ROLE
OF THE EXPERT

Opinions are not equally valuable. If we want a useful opinion on why our head throbs or our car stalls, we ask the appropriate experts. However, as we ponder accidents, we hesitate to ask the safety expert and confidently announce our own opinions perhaps after "discussing" the questions with others who know no more than we.

This contradiction stems from our failure to distinguish between *questions of knowledge* and *questions of value.* In questions of knowledge there are right and wrong answers, whereas with regard to questions of value there are differences of opinion. The layman and the expert are equally qualified to answer questions of value, but they are not equally qualified to answer questions of knowledge. For instance, the question of whether leisure time should be used in viewing operas or football games is a matter of value. But the question of whether a four-phase driver education program is as effective, less effective, or more effective than a two-phase driver education program requires expert knowledge to answer.

Stated in simple terms, *the role of the expert is not to tell people what they should want, but to tell them how they may best get what they want.* Even experts are not infallible; all may be wrong on a given issue. When experts disagree, any one answer should not be considered positive or final.

[2] Reprinted from Fred V. Hein, Dana L. Farnsworth, and Charles E. Richardson, *Living* (Glenview, Ill.: Scott, Foresman and Company, 1970), pp. 378–79, by permission of the publisher. Copyright © 1970 by Scott, Foresman and Company.

Experts in safety agree that accidents are caused and do not "just happen"; the layman who feels an accident was an event which could not have been avoided reveals his ignorance.

In the field of safety, the function of the expert is to provide accurate descriptions and analyses of accidents and to show laymen what consequences may follow each countermeasure proposal. However, experts have met with limited success when they attempt to tell people what would be best for them in a given situation. It usually takes a near-accident, an accident, or even a tragedy before people become sufficiently concerned and motivated to take overt action.

The task of the student is to learn how to recognize an expert and guide his own thinking by expert knowledge rather than by guesswork. Let us now return to objectives *1.* and *2.* listed at the beginning of the chapter to determine how well you have achieved them.

2 accident statistics: sources and problems

After reading this chapter, you should be able to:

1. *List sources of accident statistics and data.*
2. *Identify errors in collecting accident statistics.*
3. *Evaluate errors in the presentation of accident statistics.*
4. *Criticize errors in the interpretation of accident statistics.*
5. *Analyze accident statistical associations.*

The first decennial census was taken in the United States in 1790. However, it was not until after the turn of the twentieth century that accident data was collected systematically.

Accident Facts

Issued annually by the National Safety Council, *Accident Facts* now constitutes a most reliable source of nation-wide frequency for all types of accidents reported in the United States.[1] In addition to presenting annual reports on the four principal classes of accidents, *Accident Facts* presents data on rates and trends; hence this compendium provides the most reliable source for evaluating the relative efficiency of accident-

[1] *Accident Facts* may be obtained from the National Safety Council, 425 North Michigan Avenue, Chicago, Illinois 60611, for a nominal fee.

prevention agencies. The National Safety Council has been aided in the collection and interpretation of accident data by many organizations, companies, and individuals.

Other Sources of Accident Statistics

Except for statistical studies made by individual investigators which are usually limited to small samples of accident victims, the large-scale gathering of statistical data is necessarily a task of the government. At present there are several sources available for accident statistics:

1. *The Police.* Officials involved in the investigation of accidents include municipal and state police and a wide variety of sheriffs, constables, and special peace officers.

2. *Legislative Committees.* In recent years, state and national legislatures have made increasing use of their broad investigatory powers for the exploration of problems pertaining to accidents. Congressional hearings involving highway safety and consumer product safety have gained national attention.

3. *Insurance Companies.* The Metropolitan Life Insurance Company publishes a monthly publication entitled *Statistical Bulletin*. Almost every issue contains data and information pertinent to accident problems. The Traveler's Insurance Company has produced an annual booklet since 1931 (with the exception of the World War II years) containing traffic accident data and cartoon illustrations.

4. *National Center for Health Statistics.* This federal agency conducts the National Health Survey. Surveys are made of a pre-selected household sample of the entire population. Based upon the survey, an annual accidental injury total is estimated. Details of the place, nature, severity, and sources of personal injury occurring in the 2 weeks preceding the survey is gathered.

5. *State Agencies.* Organizations such as state safety councils collect, analyze, and distribute information on the incidence of accidents in their particular geographical areas.

6. *Community Agencies.* Some towns and cities also gather accident data. In addition, these agencies may serve as collecting agencies for state organizations.

7. *Other.* Data may be collected by other organizations for their own use. An elementary school or a university department of physical education may realize the need for accident reporting as an aid to accident prevention. Industry, business, and government often tabulate information concerning the frequency of accidents within their respective jurisdictions.

Problems of Statistical Analysis

An early statistician coined a phrase that has since been repeated to generations: "It's not that the figures lie—it's that the liars figure." Although deceptive figures do appear in accident statistics, it is probable that the largest number of statistical studies are compiled by those desiring to inform rather than misinform. Nevertheless, a statistic that misleads through honest error can be just as confusing as one that is deliberately constructed to misrepresent. In the following paragraphs we will discuss several sources of error found in accident statistics; these may be divided into the following groups: sources of error in *collection,* in *presentation,* and in *evaluation.*

SOURCES OF ERROR IN THE COLLECTION
OF ACCIDENT STATISTICS

Deliberate Suppression   There are several forms of suppression. One can be attributed to administrative self-protection rather than to darker motives. Keeping the accident rate down is a perennial concern of administrators. Frequently, a slightly injured worker is immediately returned to the job to keep the factory record spotless, although the injured worker should be home after the accident resting from the shock and caring for his injury.

Only a few accident statistic errors in collection result from distortions introduced deliberately or negligently. Most of these errors are either partly or totally unavoidable because there are certain problems peculiar to data-gathering. The following sources of error are highly difficult or impossible to eradicate.

Failure to Complain   Since an accident is not known until someone reports it, any statistic that purports to represent the total number of any type of accident which has taken place is necessarily an informed guess based on the addition of an estimated number of additional *unreported* accidents of the same category. Certain types of accidents tend to be reported with much greater accuracy than others. For example, deaths resulting from motor-vehicle operation are usually reported quite accurately because there are legal requirements to make such reports and great value is placed upon human life. However, motor-vehicle accidents causing less than $100 worth of damage may go unnoticed and even unreported as a result of legal stipulations and $100 deductible insurance coverage which may not require the reporting of small accidents. Even reports of damage costs may be totally in error since most estimated costs are quite subjective in nature.

Geographical Variations in the Definition of Certain Accidents
There is one obstacle hindering a uniform system of accident reporting
that will not be overcome until all jurisdictions employ similar definitions for classifying accidents. For example, a three-year-old boy is struck
by his father's automobile in the driveway while his father backs the
vehicle out of the garage. *Accident Facts* states that a motor-vehicle
accident involves an automobile in motion, whether on or off the highway
and street. Yet, a state safety council representative may categorize the
accident as a home accident and not as a motor-vehicle accident because it
occurred at home.

Differences in the Reporting of Accidents Within the Same Area   An
administrator has his biases. If a relative of his or a person with high
status has an accident, his administrator may never report it in order to
keep a record clear of any blemish which might hinder future promotions
and advancements for that person.

William E. Tarrants reported at a National Safety Congress:

> A mid-western manufacturing plant with a fairly stable injury frequency
> rate decided to hire a full-time safety engineer to see if this rate could be
> cut down. Within a short time after the safety engineer was hired, the
> injury frequency rate nearly doubled. Should we conclude that the safety
> engineer caused these accidents and quickly fire him? A closer look revealed
> that the safety engineer instituted a new accident investigation and re-
> porting system which produced more reports of disabling injuries, thus
> increasing the frequency rate.[2]

Lack of Uniformity in Collecting and Recording Techniques   Tally-
ing the number of known accidents is a considerably more complicated
process than it would seem to be. Conceivably, reports from rural areas
reveal a lower rate of actual accident occurrence than do reports from
urban areas. A motor-vehicle accident is usually witnessed whereas there
may be no witnesses to a home accident involving minor cuts or burns,
making accurate reporting more difficult.

SOURCES OF ERROR IN THE PRESENTATION
OF ACCIDENT STATISTICS

When we consider statistical data there is probably no assertion more
misleading than the frequently heard statement: "The figures speak for
themselves." Because long columns of figures convey an impression of

---

2 William E. Tarrants, "Removing the Blind Spot in Safety Education Teacher
Preparation," *School and College Safety*, National Safety Congress Transactions (Chicago: National Safety Council, 1965), p. 107.

factuality, it is essential to discuss the more common misunderstandings that arise from faulty presentation of data.

Misleading Use of Simple Sums Rather than Rates   The fact that Town *A* records 50 motor-vehicle deaths as compared with 100 reported by Town *B* does not necessarily mean that Town *B* is twice as accident-ridden as Town *A*. The reverse may be true. If Town *B* has four times the population of Town *A*, the reverse *is* true. Total accident figures do not become meaningful until they are transformed into *rates* (ratios or percentages) based on the total population under consideration. Similarly, this principle applies to changes in the incidence of accidents. Town *C*, in 1980, may report twice as many accidents as it did in 1960—yet its population may have doubled during this period. If this is true, then the accident rate remains the same.

Misleading Use of Averages and Percentages   The precaution of translating simple sums into averages and percentages does not assure the proper presentation of data; these measures can be as misleading as the raw totals. Consider the following statement: "The average number of accidents per family in the Lakeview residential area is three per year." This statement gives the impression that each family living in the Lakeview residential area has about the same number of accidents each year. This assumption may not be correct at all. A count reveals that five families live in the area. Three households report one accident, whereas the fourth family reports two accidents that year. The fifth family has a total of ten among its members. Thus the "average" figure obtained by adding the total number of accidents and dividing by five is mathematically accurate but misleading.

As the illustration demonstrates, an *average* is meaningless without information about the variation of the measures which compose it. The importance of this principle is further illustrated by an example taken from *Accident Facts*. In one year the following rates for traffic deaths were revealed for cities with populations over 1,000,000 (see Table 2–1).

On the basis of these figures we could assert that it is safer to drive a motor vehicle in Chicago than in Detroit. However, caution is still urged since a death rate based upon mileage rather than population might indicate the reverse.

Pitfalls of Graphic Presentations   For some readers, long columns of figures are not only impressing but downright intimidating. For this reason, statisticians and publicists often present their findings graphically or pictorially. Although this method presents material in quick, easy-to-comprehend form, it can also mislead the reader.

TABLE 2–1   *Motor-Vehicle Traffic Deaths per 100,000 Population for 1969 for Selected U.S. Cities*

Los Angeles	14.8
Chicago	9.7
Detroit	17.0
New York	10.5
Philadelphia	10.7
Houston	15.7

Source: Reprinted from National Safety Council, *Accident Facts* (Chicago: National Safety Council, 1970), p. 66, by permission of the Council.

SOURCES OF ERROR IN THE INTERPRETATION OF ACCIDENT STATISTICS

The "Self-evident" Conclusion   Disraeli, Mark Twain, and others have observed that there are three kinds of lies—plain lies, damned lies, and statistics. This humorous statement implies that statistics can be manipulated to support any point of view. The use of statistics, however, should not be completely dismissed, for statistics mislead and confuse only when one does not know how to interpret them. There are elaborate formulas for determining the significance and reliability of a statistic,[3] but this text offers some simple tests which the reader can apply.

In his informative and amusing book, *How To Lie with Statistics,* Darrell Huff points out a number of statistical tricks.[4] He calls attention to biased samples, meaningless averages, purposeful omissions, apple and peach comparisons, illogical correlations, the *post hoc, propter hoc* fallacy (this happened after that, therefore that caused this), the cut-off graph, the deceptive map, and the two-dimensional picture to express three-dimensional facts.

If you want to analyze a statistical statement, advises Huff, ask these questions: Who says so? How does he know? What's missing? Did somebody change the subject? Does it all make sense? He cites, among scores of amusing examples, the statement that "four times more fatalities occur on the highways at 7 P.M. than at 7 A.M." Huff says that people fail to realize that more people are killed in the evening than in the morning simply because more people are on the highways at that hour to be killed. Another amusing example of nonsense statistics is found in Table 2–2.

[3] For more information see N. M. Downie and R. W. Heath, *Basic Statistical Methods* (New York: Harper and Row, 1965), and John T. Roscoe, *Fundamental Research Statistics* (New York: Holt, Rinehart and Winston, Inc., 1969).

[4] Darrell Huff, *How To Lie with Statistics* (New York: W. W. Norton and Company, 1954).

TABLE 2–2   **Pickles Will Kill You**

Pickles will kill you: *Every pickle you eat brings you nearer to death. Amazingly the "thinking man" has failed to grasp the terrifying significance of the term "in a pickle." Although leading horticulturists have long known that* Cucumis sativas *possesses an indehiscent pepo, the pickle industry continues to expand.*

Pickles are associated with all the major diseases of the body. Eating them breeds wars and communism. They can be related to most airline tragedies. Auto accidents are caused by pickles. There exists a positive relationship between crime waves and consumption of this fruit of the cucurbit family. For example:

Nearly all sick people have eaten pickles. The effects are obviously cumulative.

99.9% of all people who die from cancer have eaten pickles.

100% of all soldiers have eaten pickles.

96.8% of all communist sympathizers have eaten pickles.

99.9% of all the people involved in air and auto accidents ate pickles within 14 days preceding the accident.

93.1% of juvenile delinquents come from homes where pickles are served frequently.

Evidence points to the long-term effects of pickle eating:

Of the people born in 1839 who later dined on pickles, there has been a 100% mortality.

All pickle-eaters born between 1849 and 1859 have wrinkled skin, have lost most of their teeth, have brittle bones and failing eyesight—if the ills of eating pickles haven't already caused their death.

Even more convincing is the report of a noted team of medical experts: rats force-fed with 20 pounds of pickles per day for 30 days developed bulging abdomens. Their appetites for WHOLESOME FOOD *were destroyed.*

In spite of all the evidence, pickle-growers and -packers continue to spread their evil. More than 120,000 acres of fertile soil are devoted to growing pickles. Our per capita yearly consumption is nearly four pounds.

Eat orchid petal soup. Practically no one has as many problems from eating orchid petal soup as they do from eating pickles.

Huff points out that many a statistic is "false on its face." "It gets by," he says, "only because the magic of numbers brings about a suspension of common sense." Huff's moral is plain: BEWARE! He characterizes the unfortunate acceptance and utilization of statistical information as follows:

The secret language of statistics, so appealing in a fact-minded culture, is employed to sensationalize, inflate, confuse, and oversimplify. Statistical methods and statistical terms are necessary in reporting the mass data of social and economic trends, business conditions, "opinion" polls, the census. But without writers who use the words with honesty and understanding and readers who know what they mean, the result can only be semantic nonsense.

In popular writing on scientific matters the abused statistic is almost crowding out the picture of the white-jacketed hero laboring overtime without time-and-a-half in an ill-lit laboratory. Like the "little dash of powder, little pot of paint," statistics are making many an important fact "look like what she ain't." A well-wrapped statistic is better than Hitler's "big lie"; it misleads, yet it cannot be pinned on you.[5]

The field of safety and accident prevention is replete with figures, statistics, numbers, and ratios. There is little literature available regarding the proper use of accident statistics. William Tarrants, at a National Safety Congress, presented information which he felt was pertinent for the safety educator. Dr. Tarrants said that:

During World War II about 375 thousand people were killed in the United States by accidents and about 408 thousand were killed in the armed forces. From these figures, it has been argued that it was not much more dangerous to be overseas in the armed forces than to be at home. A more meaningful comparison, however, would consider rates of the same age groups. This comparison would reflect adversely on the safety of the armed forces during the war—in fact, the armed forces death rate (about 12 per thousand men per year) was 15 to 20 times as high, per person per year, as the over-all civilian death rate from accidents (about 0.7 per thousand per year).

The same fallacy is noted in the widely publicized statistical appraisal which states that "Sometime during the Korean War we passed a grim milestone. One day an American soldier fell in battle. He was the 1,000,000th American soldier to die in our wars since the nation was born. A few months later the 1,000,000th American perished in a modern highway traffic accident. Our wars go back to 1776. The traffic figure starts with 1900." The article concludes that "war is dangerous business but getting from one place to another by automobile is even more dangerous." Again, we should consider rates, not numbers, and comparisons should also consider the same age groups.

Peacetime versions of the same fallacy are also common. We often hear that "off-the-job activities are more dangerous than places of work, since more accidents occur off-the-job" or that "The bedroom is the most hazardous room in the home since more injuries occur in the bedroom than any other room." Here again the originators fail to consider differences in quantity of exposure, type of exposure, age, and other influencing factors.[6]

The Confusion of Correlation with Cause   In Chapter 5 "causes" of accidents will be discussed in detail. A favorite method of searching for "causes" is to hunt for statistical associations. It is often claimed, without real justification, that there are associations and correlations between contributing factors and accidents. Students often have difficulty contrasting the association of these factors with the total situation; illustrations are given in Table 2–3 to help them overcome this difficulty. The

[5] *Ibid.*, pp. 8–9.
[6] Tarrants, pp. 107–8.

TABLE 2–3   **When Does a Percentage Indicate**
            A Statistical Association?

IF:	WE NEED TO KNOW:	BEFORE TRYING TO DECIDE:
50% of fatal accidents involve drinking drivers.	*What percent of all driving is done by drinking drivers?*	*Whether drinking drivers contribute more or less than their share of fatal accidents.*
50% of injuries to boys in the first three school grades are due to lack of knowledge.	*What percent of all boys of similar age lack safety knowledge?*	*Whether lack of knowledge is associated with school injuries to boys.*
30% of fatal accidents involve vehicles being driven too fast.	*What percent of all driving is done beyond the speed limit?*	*Whether driving too fast is correlated with fatal accidents.*
300% as many deaths occur off the job than on the job.	*What percent of time is spent both on the job and off the job?*	*Whether a worker is safer at work than elsewhere.*

central point is that a genuine association exists *only* when two things appear together *either more frequently or less frequently than would normally be expected.*

Let us return now to objectives *1.–5.* and determine how well you have achieved them.

3   *the accident problem*

After reading this chapter, you should be able to:

1. *Describe the extent of accident occurrence.*
2. *Define the nine types and four principal classes of accidents.*
3. *Analyze the geographical distribution of accidents.*
4. *Identify the general characteristics of the accident "victim."*
5. *Give examples of the social and economic consequences of accidents.*

The Extent of Accident Occurrence

Reading statistics can be quite dull. Reading accident statistics may be repulsive and gory as well. However, reading statistics of any kind only tells us where and how accidents happened, but not why. Let us consider some general accident statistics.

Every year in this country approximately 115,000 deaths are reported by the National Safety Council. This averages out to one death every five minutes.[1] About 11 million injuries are reported annually. Disabling injuries are not reported on a nationwide basis, therefore the total numbers of injuries are estimates and should not be compared from year to year. However, the number of work injuries tabulated tends to be quite accurate because there is good reporting and an established defini-

[1] National Safety Council, *Accident Facts* (Chicago: National Safety Council, 1970), p. 20.

tion of a disabling injury. In contrast, the total number of nondisabling injuries treated at home, in doctors' offices, or in emergency hospital rooms is unknown.

The accident picture in the United States is grim; yet it is fair to assume that without organized safety efforts and safety education, America's accident record would be even more shocking than it is. Following heart disease, cancer, and strokes, accidents are the fourth principal cause of death in the United States. Accidents are the leading cause of death among those persons aged one to thirty-seven years.[2]

We often think of accidents only when they are catastrophes because these events make newspaper headlines. From a statistical point of view, a catastrophe is an accident in which five or more lives are lost.[3] It is significant that a very small percentage of accident catastrophes occur as a result of natural forces such as floods, hurricanes, tornadoes, and earthquakes (See Fig. 3–1). Rather, the majority of newspaper headline catastrophes are caused by some kind of human failure which results in airplane crashes, mine cave-ins, explosions, etc. However, the record of national catastrophes reveals that relatively few lives are lost in this way when contrasted with the total number of deaths resulting from other types of unspectacular, unpublished accidents.

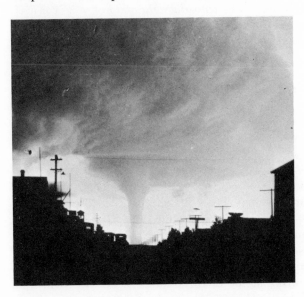

FIGURE 3–1 Tornadoes occur in many parts of the world and in all 50 states. They are the most violent type of weather condition; however, the hurricane is the most destructive. Reproduced courtesy of the National Oceanic and Atmospheric Administration.

2 All statistical references in this book are from the National Safety Council publication, *Accident Facts*, 1970.

3 Metropolitan Life Insurance Company, *Statistical Bulletin* (New York: Metropolitan Life Insurance Company, August 1970), p. 8.

Surveys of Accidents
Among the General Public

The National Health Survey, conducted by the National Center for Health Statistics, is a survey of households concerned with collecting the number of injuries sustained by household members during the two weeks prior to the survey interview. (It should be noted that other health information is also surveyed.) The total number of injuries is then estimated for the entire United States based upon these findings from approximately 40,000 households. We realize that differences in definition produce different injury totals when we compare the results of the National Health Survey with the totals presented by the National Safety Council.

An examination of accident injury data gathered from the general population suggests the following conclusions:

1. Estimates of the number of accidents based solely on the data of deaths or reported injuries are incomplete.
2. Data derived from these sources point out the need for a standard accident definition and reporting system.

The question of definition—and *who does the defining*—is a crucial one. For example, one may never detect or report the housewife who burns her fingers. This type of incident occurs commonly in daily living and illustrates how large numbers of accidents remain unknown.

Regardless of the error and incompleteness of accident data, we can conclude that there is definitely an immense loss from accidents.

The Anatomy of Accidents
in the United States

The accidents reported in *Accident Facts* are categorized into nine separate types and four principal classes. In view of the differing definitions of accidents used by various agencies, this categorization represents an impressive achievement; without it and the National Health Survey, an overall estimate or source of accident rates would not exist. Because of its importance in providing standarized definitions of accident types, an adaption of the categorization found in *Accident Facts* is provided in Table 3–1 on page 21.

Accident Facts lists the principal classes of accidents as motor-vehicle, work, home, and public. Table 3–2 (page 22) defines each of the four classes. Each class is then subdivided into accident types. For example, public accident types are listed.

TABLE 3–1   **Types of Accidents**

ALL ACCIDENTS   *The term "accidents" includes most deaths and injuries from violence, but specifically excludes homicides, committed and attempted suicides and deaths and injuries in war operations.*

MOTOR-VEHICLE ACCIDENTS   *Includes those accidents involving mechanically or electrically powered highway-transport vehicles in motion (except those on rails), both on and off the highway or street.*

FALLS   *Includes falls from one level to another or on the same level, except falls in or from railway-, road-, water-, or air-transport vehicles, or those occurring in cataclysms.*

DROWNING   *Includes all drownings (work and nonwork) in boat accidents and those resulting from swimming, playing in the water, or falling in. Excludes drownings in floods and other cataclysms.*

FIRES, BURNS, AND DEATHS ASSOCIATED WITH FIRES   *Includes those accidents from fires, burns, and from injuries in conflagrations—such as asphyxiation, falls, and being struck by falling objects. Excludes burns from hot objects or liquids.*

FIREARMS   *Includes firearm accidents in recreational activities or on home premises and a small number (less than 3 percent) from explosions of dynamite, bombs, grenades, etc. Excludes accidents in war operations.*

POISONING BY SOLIDS AND LIQUIDS   *Includes those accidents resulting from medicines, as well as from commonly recognized poisons. Mushroom and shellfish poisoning are included, but poisoning from spoiled foods— botulism, etc.—is classified as disease.*

MACHINERY ACCIDENTS   *Includes those accidents involving all types of machinery. Nearly half occur on farms in the course of work; of these, approximately three-fourths involve tractors. About one-third occur in industry. Five percent occur in the home.*

POISONING BY GASES AND VAPORS   *Principally carbon monoxide due to incomplete combustion, involving cooking stoves, heating equipment and standing motor vehicles. Excludes accidents in conflagrations, or associated with transport vehicles in motion.*

ALL OTHER TYPES   *Most important types included are: inhalation or ingestion of food or other objects, mechanical suffocation, air transportation, blow by falling object, electric current, railroad, excessive heat or cold, cataclysm.*

Source: Adapted from the National Safety Council, *Accident Facts* (Chicago: National Safety Council, 1970), pp. 6–7, by permission of the Council.

1. Falls
2. Drowning
3. Firearms
4. Fires, burns, and deaths associated with fires
5. Air transport
6. Water transport
7. Railroad
8. Other transport
9. All other public accidents

TABLE 3–2   Classes of Accidents

MOTOR-VEHICLE   *Includes those accidents involving mechanically or electrically powered highway-transport vehicles in motion (except those on rails), both on and off the highway or street.*

WORK   *Includes those accidents which arise out of and in the course of gainful work, except that (1) work injuries to domestic servants, and (2) injuries occurring in connection with farm chores, are classified as home injuries.*

HOME   *Includes those accidents in the home and on home premises to occupants, guests, and trespassers. Also includes domestic servants but excludes other persons working on home premises.*

PUBLIC   *Includes those accidents in public places or places used in a public way, not involving motor vehicles. Most sports and recreation deaths are included. Excludes accidents in the course of employment.*

Source: Adapted from National Safety Council, *Accident Facts* (Chicago: National Safety Council, 1970), pp. 42, 72, 82, 97, by permission of the Council.

Estimates of the Cost of Accidents

Reliable estimates of the overall cost per annum of accidents in the United States are difficult to make, and those who have investigated the problem will probably conclude that even approximate figures would be inaccurate.

We can compare accident costs to an iceberg—only a small portion appears above water that we can actually see and measure. The indirect and hidden costs form the bottom of the iceberg, the part below water that is not easily measured. Like the iceberg, hidden costs of accidents are not visible on the surface but they are there just the same. Examples of hidden costs are among those listed in Table 3–3.

The Geographical Distribution of Accidents in the United States

REGIONAL ACCIDENT RATES

Rates of reported accidents vary widely from one region to another. In accidental death rates, the Middle Atlantic region ranks lowest. The Rocky Mountain region has the highest rate of accidental deaths. Various explanations.could be offered for these wide variations, but they would probably still not account for all the variations found.

RURAL–URBAN VARIATIONS

Accident death rates tend consistently to increase with greater density of population. The difference in rates between the most densely populated and the least densely populated communities is sizable.

RURAL ACCIDENT RATES

For reporting purposes, *Accident Facts* classifies areas with at least 2,500 inhabitants as "rural." Because they are incomplete or not tabulated, reports from rural areas probably reveal a lower rate of actual accident occurrence than do reports from urban areas.

Interpreting Rural–Urban Accident Distribution

The apparently consistent relationship between population density and accidental death rates leads us to conclude that the higher the population concentration, the higher the accident rate (See Fig. 3–2). When the urban centers are grouped in descending order of size, the accident

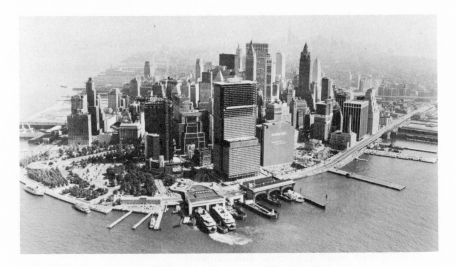

FIGURE 3–2   A view of the New York City skyline—Lower Manhattan (Wall Street). Accident death rates tend to increase with population density. Reproduced courtesy of the New York Convention and Visitors Bureau; photo by Allen Green taken from a Hel-Aire Copter.

rate decreases. Difficulties arise, however, with this general explanation:

1. Urban centers of similar size but in different regions of the country show great variation in their accident rates.
2. Even within the same geographical region, the rates do not always decline according to declining size of population.
3. Among cities the same size and within the same region, there are often significant variations in accident rates which can only be accounted for in terms of factors specific to the particular cities.

The last explanation brings us closer to the core of the accident problem.

General Characteristics of
The Accident Victim

The "typical" accident victim exists only as a vague abstraction created from statistical figures. Nevertheless, statistics enable us to say:

1. Most accident victims are males. After the first year of life, males have more accidents than females, at all age levels.
2. Most accident victims are young. Accidents are the leading cause of death for persons aged one to 37 years; however, the rate for accidental deaths is highest for those under one and over 65 years of age.
3. Most accident victims reside in an urban center; the Rocky Mountain region of the United States has the highest accident rate.
4. Most accidental deaths occur in a motor vehicle but most injuries occur in the home.
5. Most accidents occur to the victim in a cyclical nature reaching peaks in frequency on a certain day and at a particular time in the year.

As we discussed in Chapter 2, finding a way to make facts talk without having them say more than they actually do presents a real problem.

Social and Economic Consequences
of Accidents

Accidents produce consequences of grave importance. Table 3–3 presents in brief form some social and economic implications of accidents. We should consider the serious consequences of accidents in terms of

TABLE 3–3 **Some Social and Economic Consequences**
of Accidents

SOCIAL	ECONOMIC
1. *Grief over the loss of loved ones*	1. *Wage losses*
2. *Denial of education*	2. *Medical and hospital fees*
3. *Lack of guidance for children*	3. *Property damage*
4. *Psychological effects of a change in standard of living*	4. *Production loss for employer*
5. *Physical handicaps causing re-adjustment, retraining, and job placement*	5. *Loss of earning capability*
6. *Major cause of death*	6. *Rise in insurance premium cost and liability payments*
7. *Psychic damages affecting behavior*	7. *Loss of profit on idle machinery damaged or awaiting repairs*
8. *Embarrassment and lost pride*	8. *Work stoppage for assisting the injured, curiosity, cleaning up, etc. which results in non-productive wages paid to non-injured*
9. *Inconvenience*	9. *Need for working mother*
10. *Interpersonal relationships affected adversely from anger, resentment, etc.*	10. *Loss of talent*

their disruptive effects on the home, on the family, and on employment.
The notions of "life years lost" and "working years lost" are helpful in
gauging the magnitude of the accident problem. Table 3–4 shows us that
back in 1945, accidental deaths were responsible for a greater loss of
working years in the country than were deaths from those diseases listed
in Table 3–4.

TABLE 3–4 **Estimated Number of Working Years**
Lost in the U.S. in 1945
As a Result of Death from Various Causes

CAUSE OF DEATH	WORKING YEARS LOST (THOUSANDS)	PERCENTAGE OF TOTAL DEATHS
Accidents	1,980	12.6
Heart disease	1,892	12.0
Pneumonia	1,274	8.1
Cancer	1,155	7.3
Tuberculosis	1,144	7.3
Nephritis (kidney disease)	484	3.1
Cerebrovascular disease	465	3.0

Source: Reprinted from "the Unsleeping Dragon," *World Health,* The
Magazine of the World Health Organization (June 1967), p. 7, by permission
of the World Health Organization.

Let us return now to objectives *1.–5.* and determine how well you have
achieved them.

4 *philosophical implications*

After reading this chapter, you should be able to:

1. *Explain reasons for death and suffering.*
2. *List reasons for avoiding accidents and prolonging life.*
3. *Summarize basic beliefs held by safety authorities.*
4. *Define risk and identify the types of risk-taking.*
5. *Give examples of safety issues.*

The types of accident problems discussed in this book fall into two main categories: those caused by natural forces and those which are the result of man's action. Both can result in suffering or death. Examples of those accidents which occur from natural causes are: a fatal shipwreck caused by a storm; death in the (frozen) north by freezing due to insufficient food and clothing; a hurricane that causes death from flooding and other damage; a tidal wave that strikes the West Coast causing death to hundreds; death from a grizzly bear attack on hikers in Yellowstone National Park; death from a rattlesnake bite in southern Texas.

Many justify these natural calamities by maintaining that they impel us to overcome them, and teach us how to live in the world. For example, the tornado teaches us to build storm cellars for protection and to set up weather observation points for advance warning. The tidal wave that struck the Hawaiian Islands a few years ago caused great devastation of life and property and taught the Hawaiians certain lessons; now when tidal waves strike the Islands, very few, if any, lives are lost. Men, then, are forced by circumstances to devise ways of signaling the danger before it arrives.

Certainly, one of the most universal and perplexing problems facing mankind is the existence of suffering. Is suffering a punishment for laws broken? Do the innocent suffer with the guilty? Can man grow through suffering? Is suffering necessary for greatness? (Most great men have suffered.)

Great works of literature often give us insight into the purpose of suffering and death in life. For example, we see suffering in the book of Job in the Bible, and the suggestion of growth through suffering in the life of Hester Prynne in Hawthorne's *The Scarlet Letter.* "The Lament" by Anton Chekhov presents two universal human qualities: the need to share sorrow and the difficulty of finding anyone sympathetic to share it with. Luigi Pirandello's "War" is a story of the struggle between the mind's abilty to reason away sorrow and the emotions' tendency to burst forth beyond the control of reason. "Compensation" by Ralph Waldo Emerson makes some profound explorations into suffering. Emerson tells us that in every triumph there is defeat, and in every defeat triumph; in every gain there is loss, and in every loss gain; in every pleasure there is pain, and in every pain pleasure; and all experiences of success and failure, health and sickness, happiness and sorrow balance themselves out, which he calls "compensation." William Wordsworth's poem "Michael" depicts the developing greatness of his central character through his suffering—which dignifies him.

The experience of death comes to every man, for sooner or later, we all must die. This experience affects us in two ways: (1) we die young and bring sorrow to family and friends, or (2) we live long and feel sorrow as family and friends die. Man's reactions to death are well-portrayed in works by poets, dramatists and novelists such as Hemingway's *For Whom the Bell Tolls* or Miller's *Death of a Salesman.* "The Death of a Dauphin" by Alphonse Daudet, for example, shows us the universality of death, whereas poems like Edward Fitzgerald's translation of "The Rubaiyat of Omar Khayyam," James Thomson's "The City of Dreadful Night," and Robinson Jeffers' "May–June 1940" reflect a negative attitude towards death. Poems expressing positive views are William Shakespeare's "Sonnet 146," John Donne's "Death Be Not Proud," William Wordsworth's "We Are Seven," as well as "Prospice" and "Rabbi Ben Ezra" by Robert Browning.

The second type of problem consists of those accidents which are the direct result of man's behavior. Three factors seem to explain suffering caused by human behavior.

1. We have made great scientific advancements because we can rely on

the basic law and order of our physical world—two and two always make four and not five. The solar system moves in mathematically correct orbits, enabling us to land a man on the moon (See Fig. 4–1). The earth's gravitational pull determines that what we throw into the air must be pulled back to the earth; this always happens—even though the object might be a car that plunges off a mountain road taking the occupants to their deaths.

2. Man is a free agent. He is prevented from doing what he wants because there are limits set upon him by the environment in which he lives, as well as various social circumstances and limitations of the physical body. Being a free agent, however, means that he can do what he pleases, but will suffer the consequences of his actions—good or bad.

3. What one person does may vitally affect his neighbors because human lives are intermingled. When automobile accident insurance premiums rise, the owner of a car with no accident record becomes alarmed. After all, he is paying for others' accidents. Thus, other people's behavior affects him. When an automobile crosses through the freeway median guardrail and crashes into another car, killing its occupants, it is obvious that others have been affected by this stranger's actions and behavior.

Dying and death are events from which none of us escape. We can

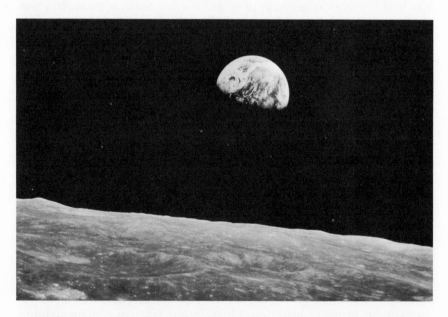

FIGURE 4–1   This view of the rising earth greeted astronauts of Apollo 8 as they came from behind the moon (the sunset terminator bisects Africa). Reproduced courtesy of the National Aeronautics and Space Administration.

postpone death, gain reprieves from it, but ultimately we must die. Many people react to these statements by feeling there is something morbid in thinking about death. They comment, "I'm interested in life, not death." Is this not a form of ostrich behavior to avoid one of the essential realities of life?

The critical question is not the dichotomy of life and death but rather how each one of us reacts to the knowledge that death is inevitable. Throughout man's history, the concept of death has been at the core of our religious and philosophical thought and thus affects our outlook toward daily living.

Contradictions arise about the existence of death. Death is viewed by some as a "wall," the ultimate personal disaster, whereas others regard death as a "doorway," a point in time on the way to eternity. However, while we are living, we should do all we can to preserve our lives.

Reasons for Safety

In the previous section we examined ideas pertaining to suffering and death which attempt to soften the "sting of death." Several reasons for avoiding accidents which produce injury and death are:

1. To avoid pain
2. To avoid inconvenience
3. To avoid material loss
4. To maintain a good record
5. To protect life
6. To preserve talent (see Table 4–1)
7. To avoid other social and economic consequences. (See Table 3–3 p. 25.)

The period of greatest achievement for artists, authors, scientists, and scholars averages just under 50 years of age, reports Thorndike. Sorenson supports Thorndike's "masterpiece age" by reporting that most scholars and scientists do their best work at about fifty years of age with a variance within ten-year periods before and after fifty.[1]

---

[1] Harold S. Diehl, *Healthful Living* (New York: McGraw-Hill Book Company, 1968), p. 8.

TABLE 4–1   **Missing Contributions**

What does society lose by the premature impairment or death of genius? Can society ever measure that intangible potential that was never realized? What might the world have gained by improving the vitality and length of life of persons with great abilities?

NAME	PARTIAL CONTRIBUTIONS OR IDENTIFICATION	AGE AT DEATH	APPROXIMATE NUMBER OF YEARS LOST
Louis Braille	Devised braille system of reading for the blind	43	27
John M. Burnham	Designer of the submarines Nautilus, Seawolf, and Skate	40	30
Edwin J. Cohn	Medical research authority (gamma globulin, etc.)	59	11
Stephen Crane	Journalist, novelist, poet	29	41
Guy de Maupassant	Writer of almost 300 short stories and novels	43	27
Enrico Fermi	Nuclear physicist	53	17
Eugene Gardner	Atomic physicist	37	33
John C. Glover	A.A.U. 100-yard swimming champion, 1955	22	48
Joseph G. Hamilton	Pioneer in atomic medicine	49	21
Thomas J. "Stonewall" Jackson	Military leader	39	31
John Keats	Poet	26	44
Joseph W. Kennedy	Discoverer of plutonium	40	30
Edward Arthur Milne	One of the world's great mathematicians	54	16
Wolfgang Amadeus Mozart	One of the world's renowned composers	35	35
Takashi Nagai	Medical and radiation scientist	43	27
Edgar Allen Poe	Author and poet	39	31
Raphael Sanzio	Painter	37	33
Edward R. Stettinius	Diplomat and Secretary of State	49	21
Robert Louis Stevenson	Novelist	44	26
Johann Strauss	Composer of more than 150 of the world's most beautiful waltzes	45	25
Henry David Thoreau	Author and naturalist	45	25

LOST IN THIS GROUP ALONE, 599 YEARS OF GENIUS IN GIVEN FIELDS.

Source: Data courtesy of O.E. Byrd, Stanford University; Dick Hayden, from an unpublished manuscript.

Summary of Basic "Core" Beliefs

Today, most safety educators and specialists are in agreement with the following basic statements:

1. Safety is not an end in itself; it is just a means to a more productive life. "Safety First" is a poor slogan.
2. Safety involves more than just avoiding accidents.
3. Safety is a relative thing and is extremely difficult to define. It varies from day to day which implies that a person is at different levels of safety every day of his life.
4. Safety is a many-sided subject which draws upon interdisciplinary fields for its approach and content.
5. Accidents are caused and thus are preventable.
6. There are no such things as chance and luck. Luck and chance are names for unrecognized causes.
7. Human life has value and should be preserved.
8. "Life at its best is taking risks for things worthwhile."
9. Safety education reduces the risks in living.

Risk

Risk or danger is inherent in life. From an optimistic point of view, life is an adventure and man is continually pushing into new endeavors which are frequently dangerous (see Fig. 4–2). For example, exhilarating

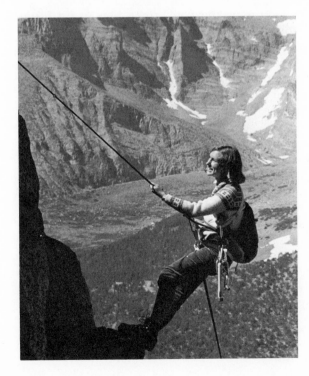

FIGURE 4–2 What may be risky for some may not be for others. Reproduced courtesy of Kent and Donna Dannen. Photo by Kent and Donna Dannen.

leisure-time activities such as mountain climbing, motor cycling, para-
chuting, scuba diving, and snowmobiling are probably adventuresome
enough to attract millions of participants annually. Yet, in the opinion
of other millions of non-participants, the sports enthusiasts of these
activities are labeled dare-devils or even "crazy."

Let us examine the term "risk" as a very important concept in relation
to safe behavior.

> Most people tend to use the term *risk* with two meanings. First, they mean
> the inherent danger in a situation. Usually the situation or action is called
> risky, implying in a mixed way both that there is danger and that the actor
> is behaving with likelihood of accident or injury as a result of this behavior.
> But if no one is actually behaving, people talk about the absolute risk of a
> situation. Secondly, people talk about a person's taking risk, implying that
> he has deliberately entered a dangerous situation. There is little implica-
> tion here that the "risk" is attributable to the situation—more to the
> person's behaving in this admittedly dangerous situation.
>   I propose that we use two words which will separate these meanings more
> clearly. They are "hazard" and "risk." "Hazard" will be objective danger
> or likelihood of failure, and "risk" will be subjective estimate of hazard.
>   The usage proposed—that is, hazard = danger, and risk = estimated
> hazard—can become formalized easily . . . .[2]

Dr. Fox indicates that most of us know only three types of risk-takers:
(1) "those who are perfectly aware of danger and act with eyes wide open,"
(2) "those who are only partially aware of the hazards," and (3) "those who
are ignorant of the hazards, assuming complete safety." Fox indicates
other classes of risk-takers in addition to the three commonly named
above: (1) those "not thinking about hazard," (2) "those who take no
risk," (3) those who believe there is "no hazard," (4) those who deliberately appraise the hazard and (5) those who believe they are invul-
nerable.[3]

Why people intentionally take risks varies with each individual. Risk-
taking is influenced by an evaluation of the odds—is there enough potential gain to assume the hazard? Among the "rewards" for successful
risk-taking are saving time, gaining status, experiencing a thrill, satisfy-
ing our egos, and punishing ourselves and others.

Risk, then, is a relative thing. What may be risky to one person may be
an everyday event to another. The margin of safety varies from person to
person and even changes for the same person at different times and in
different locations. In some risk-taking activities the margin of safety is

---

[2] Bernard H. Fox, "Discussion," *Behavioral Approaches to Accident Research,* (New
York: Association for the Aid of Crippled Children, 1961), p. 50.

[3] *Ibid.,* pp. 52–53.

the same for all. For example, in sky diving or mountain climbing, risk is obviously relative to the skill and experience of the participant—less skill increases the hazard. However, in Russian roulette with a six-chamber revolver and only one bullet, the margin of safety is the same for all participants—there are no experts.

Most societies have their risk-takers. Whether they be Vikings or astronauts, they have received a hero's reward in victory or in death. Sports such as bullfighting, boxing, sports car and motorcycle racing, ice hockey, football, surfing, mountain climbing, sky diving, scuba diving, and snow skiing all involve risks. Contemporary "heroes" are among the participants in these sport activities.

Issues in Safety

There are differing points of view with regard to specific topics and concerns in safety. These issues should be studied because they:

1. Need resolving or answering.
2. Are seldom found in textbooks because they are recent.
3. Can and do affect people.
4. Are interesting and provocative.

Listed below are some controversial issues related to safety:

1. The school safety patrol.
2. Driver and traffic safety education.
3. Firearm and ammunition registration.
4. Small vs. large cars—which are safer?
5. Football, boxing, and javelin throwing in the high schools.
6. Required safety equipment in automobiles.
7. Required motorcycle helmet laws.
8. Alcohol tests and implied consent laws.
9. The use of snowmobiles.

Certainly this textbook will not attempt to resolve the above issues or any others. However, the reader will recall from Chapter 1 the difference between knowledge judgments and value judgments which will aid him in answering questions with regard to the problem of accidents and safety.

A high regard for safety competes occasionally with time, status, and group pressures, personality shortcomings, courage, adventure, and other factors. A concern for safety enables us to choose between experiences that are unproductive, absurd, and even stupid, and those that enrich our lives, making them interesting and worthwhile. Our aim should be safety *for* rather than safety *from*.

Let us return now to objectives *1.–5.* and determine how well you have achieved them.

5 concepts of accident causation and countermeasures

After reading this chapter, you should be able to:

1. *Explain the multiple-cause concept.*
2. *Describe and appraise epidemiology as a method for determining causation.*
3. *Identify the etiology and countermeasures for an accident type.*
4. *Define and evaluate the concept of accident proneness.*
5. *Point out the relationship between behavior and the models associated with it.*
6. *Explain modes of influencing behavior by giving examples in safety of each mode.*

Multiple-Cause Concept

Accidents generally result from a combination of closely interwoven factors. Let us consider these factors in detail.

Each of the factors which contributes to an accident is *a* cause, whereas *the* cause is the combination of these factors, each of which is necessary but none of which is sufficient by itself. A *factor* is any condition or action accompanying an accident whether it contributes to the accident or not. A contributing *cause* is a factor without which the accident would not have happened. Therefore, a cause is always a factor, but a factor is not always a cause.[1] Each cause, if it truly contributes to an accident, is an

[1] Automotive Safety Foundation, *A Resource Curriculum Guide in Driver and Traffic Safety Education* (Washington, D.C.: Automotive Safety Foundation, 1970), p. 75.

equally important factor in that accident, but could be identified as being distant, intermediate, or immediate in its relation to an accident.

The accident victim may "get away with" violations for years because all the other essential ingredients for an accident were not present. However, this does not guarantee that an accident would not occur the first time a violation is committed.

Too often the event directly preceding an accident is labeled the cause. The multiple-cause concept refutes this.

Epidemiology of Accidents

"Epidemic" literally means "in or among people" and thus "common to, or affecting at the same time, many in a community." Formerly, epidemiology was defined as the medical science dealing with epidemics. It was most often found in public health programs which dealt with infectious and communicable diseases. However, heart disease, cancer (noninfectious diseases), and accidents have also been studied by the epidemiologist. The epidemiological approach to accident prevention has received much attention in recent literature. Dr. John Gordon[2] (probably the first to use the epidemiological approach to the accident problem) and others emphasize the importance of viewing accidents as a public health problem because they play an increasingly significant role as a cause of death. They also stress the fact that this problem should be treated in the same way, with the same methods used in the epidemiological approach to other public health problems.

The epidemiologist usually collects information on three sets of factors which interact to cause the problem: (1) host or human factors, (2) agent factors, and (3) environmental factors. For example, if a child falls from a swing and strikes her head on the ground, we would call the child the host, the ground the agent which produced injury, and the location and design of the swing the environment. This approach to accident study leads us to conclude that it takes a combination of factors (as was discussed in the previous section) to cause an accident.

Host factors include a consideration of age, sex, marital status, race, and physical condition. Agent factors are not always as obvious. The agent may be described as the object most closely associated with the accident such as faulty brakes or a loaded gun. Or it may be those things which inflict injury such as glass, poison, or fire (See Fig. 5–1). The type of accident—motor vehicle, fall, drowning, etc.—is a third agent classifica-

---

[2] John E. Gordon, "The Epidemiology of Accidents," *American Journal of Public Health,* XXXIX (April 1949), 504–15.

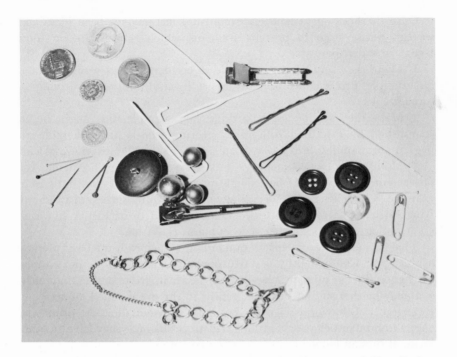

FIGURE 5–1 *Things children swallow. Reproduced courtesy of New York State Health News, a monthly publication of the New York State Department of Health; photo by M. Dixson.*

tion. The automobile can then be the "agent of the accident" (type of accident), or it can be the "agent of the injury" (steering wheel column spears the driver's chest), or it may be the "agent of circumstance" (faulty brakes). Environmental factors include: time, weather, seasons, location or place, and geography.

An epidemiological approach was used in the study of off-duty motor-vehicle accidents by military personnel. Study revealed that the accidents were not related to long-distance weekend driving, but to short-distance driving around the military base, usually in the late evening or early morning hours. The high-rate accident group was identified as young, unmarried, enlisted men in search of recreational activity which usually included drinking. In addition, a high proportion of accidents occurred on a few particular sections of highway. As a result of the study recommendations, military police patrolled the high-incident sections of highway. The countermeasures that were put in effect resulted in a 42 percent decrease in the accident rate.[3]

[3] Ross A. McFarland and Roland C. Moore, "The Epidemiology of Accidents," in *Accident Prevention,* ed. Maxwell N. Halsey (New York: McGraw-Hill Book Company, 1961), p. 22.

Once the host, agent, and environmental factors have been identified, we can devise steps to prevent accidents which concentrate on those factors in order to:

1. Make the "host" less susceptible to accidents. This would involve, for example, driver education, abstinence from alcohol while driving, or tornado alerts.

2. Make the "agent" less hazardous. For example, this might be accomplished by installing collapsible steering wheels and inflatable air bags in automobiles, break-away road signs, or safety lenses in eye glasses.

3. Modify the environment so it is less conducive to accidents. Improvement of freeways by better lighting and additional guardrails is an example. The science of epidemiology has been quite successful in identifying causative factors of disease. When applied to accidents, however, epidemiology describes rather than explains causation.

That accidents are a manifestation of human behavior is a basic premise of this book. Consequently, as stated previously, accidents do not happen by chance. Just as human behavior may result in crime and delinquency, so it may be that similar behavior results in the event called an accident. Regrettably, behavioral scientists have not devoted their attention and efforts to human behavior and the accident problem as they have to other forms of human behavior and their consequences.

Etiology and Countermeasures

Dr. William Haddon, Jr. introduced a conceptual model for the U.S. Government's program to curtail traffic accident losses. Use of the model may be extended to other accident types as well. The model consists of three phases which lead to an accident.

The *first phase* (pre-event, pre-accident, or pre-contact) consists of the many factors which determine whether or not an accident will take place. Elements that cause people and physical and/or chemical forces to move into undesirable interaction are included here.

The *second phase* (event, accident, or contact) begins when physical and/or chemical forces exert themselves unfavorably upon people and/or property.

The *third phase* (post-event, post-accident, or post-contact) involves salvaging people and/or property after the damage has been done.

We can develop a matrix by using both the three phases and the three factors involved in epidemiology (host, agent, environment). Categorizing contributing causal factors of an accident type may indicate why accident losses occur. Countermeasures for reducing accident losses can be formed by constructing a second matrix utilizing the same phases and factors.

Tables 5–1 and 5–2 give an example of contributing factors and their countermeasures for one accident type—discarded or abandoned refrigerators. Of course, not all of the contributing factors or countermeasures are given. Remember that this framework can be applied to most accident types.

Accident Proneness

There is a difference between accident repetitiveness and accident proneness. An accident repeater is an individual who has more than one accident of the same type. Accident proneness describes a person who has more accidents than others. Several authorities list personality traits characteristic of the accident prone. However, research indicates that there is no such thing as one type of accident prone person. Rather, each individual develops a range of behavior; some of the behavior is safe and

TABLE 5–1 **Contributing Factors**

Accident type: *Discarded or Abandoned Refrigerators*

Factors / Phases	Host (human)	Agent	Environment
Pre-event	Children are attracted to "playthings"—refrigerator becomes a hiding place, playhouse, and/or jail	Refrigerators can contain a child or several children (one case reported that 5 children suffocated together.)	Refrigerators are abandoned in remote areas (i.e., junkyards) or are temporarily in disuse (as in empty apartments or those in the process of defrosting)
Event	Inability for human to exist in oxygen deficit environment for over 10–15 minutes	Children are trapped in a sealed, "airtight" heavily insulated compartment	Abandoned refrigerators are usually in remote areas away from people who might observe children playing in or around them
Post-event	Oxygen deficit by victims	Child not visible unless the refrigerator door is open	Difficulty in locating the missing child by searchers

Source: Adapted from William Haddon, Jr., "A Logical Framework for Categorizing Highway Safety Phenomena and Activity," *Journal of Trauma* (in press, 1971), by permission of the author.

TABLE 5–2   **Countermeasures**

Accident type: *Discarded or Abandoned Refrigerators*

Factors / Phases	Host (human)	Agent	Environment
Pre-event	*Tell children to stay away from discarded refrigerators because they are not "playthings" and they can kill*	*Manufacturers install permanent trays in refrigerators which don't allow room for children to crawl into them*	*Imposed penalties for discarding refrigerators without removing hinges and door*
Event	*If a child is missing, a first place to look is in refrigerators*	*Manufacturers install an interior wall section which a child's force can puncture to allow ventilation*	*Manufacturers install an alerting device which would indicate occupancy and use (light or buzzer)*
Post-event	*Resuscitation training for parents and older children*	*Escape worthiness, (i.e., door can be opened from within by a force of 5 pounds)*	*A first place to look for missing children is in refrigerators*

Source: Adapted from William Haddon, Jr., "A Logical Framework for Categorizing Highway Safety Phenomena and Activity," *Journal of Trauma* (in press, 1971), by permission of the author.

some unsafe, depending also on the environmental hazards to which he is exposed. Dr. Frederick McGuire sums up current thinking on accident proneness probably as well as anyone:

> [A]ccident proneness *does* exist in some people for at least short periods of time, exists in others for relatively long periods of time, and is in both instances predictable if properly measured at the right time.[4]

Suffice it to say that the accident prone concept is greatly misunderstood and is often misused as an explanation for all cases of repeated accidents. In other words, if an individual has one or more accidents, it does not mean he is accident prone. In rejecting previous emphasis placed on accident proneness, we do not exclude the important role played by personal factors in accident occurrence.

Again, accident proneness refers to relatively consistent characteristics

[4] Frederick L. McGuire, "A Typology of Accident Proneness," *Behavioral Research in Highway Safety,* I (January 1970), 32.

which make the person more susceptible to accidents. Data show that there are such people, but their number is small and their contribution to the total accident problem is slight.

Almost all people have accidents. When a person has difficulty adjusting to the environment, he is referred to as temporarily accident prone or accident susceptible. However, if one is susceptible, it does not mean an accident will inevitably occur.

Imitation

There are several ways in which behavior is influenced. Some of the most obvious agents which deliberately attempt to induce specific behavior are television commercials, public schools, and parental discipline.

Behavior is also strongly influenced by what we learn through imitating others. "Do as I say and not as I do" is a saying that reflects the fact that people sometimes learn more from imitation than we would like to admit. A little girl does not dress up in her mother's clothes and high heels because she has been taught to do so; she is doing what she has seen her mother do.

A person's attitudes and behavior are strongly influenced by the people with whom he associates. The power of social influence is illustrated by an experimental situation in which 90 students with differing degrees of thirst were faced with a sign over a drinking fountain which read, "Do not use this fountain." The students had been told that the experiment they were to take part in was a study of taste preferences rather than a study of social influence. Differing degrees of thirst were induced by asking the students to eat varying numbers of crackers, some treated with hot sauce. After eating the crackers, the subjects were asked to step into the hall for a few moments on the pretext that the next part of the "taste experiment" was not yet ready to start.

While they were in the hall, the students saw the water fountain and the sign prohibiting its use. One group of students observed someone else who did not conform to the prohibition. The other group of students, a control group, was not exposed to anyone else's reaction to the sign.

The critical question in the experiment was: could someone else exert any influence on the decisions and actions of the individual? The finding indicated that when students saw someone else violate the prohibition, they were more likely to drink from the fountain themselves than were the students who observed conforming behavior.[5]

Research on imitation tells us that we must behave in the way we want

[5] D. L. Kimbrell and R. R. Blake, "Motivational Factors in the Violation of a Prohibition," *Journal of Abnormal and Social Psychology*, LVI (1958), 132–33.

our children and students to behave. It confirms the fact that when your behavior is hypocritical, the teaching is less effective than if you practice what you teach.[6]

The significance of imitation is well documented. With regard to the tendency to imitate and its effects on safety, Michigan State University researchers say that fathers with numerous traffic convictions tend to have sons who have numerous traffic convictions. Fathers with no convictions tend to have sons with no convictions. How a young man drives seems to be influenced more by his family than by driver education or the actions of police and courts.[7]

There are other methods of influencing behavior which vary in effectiveness with the process of imitation. For example, exhortation, often used in encouraging accident prevention, has seldom been very successful in influencing behavior. Most of us would rather learn by example than by being told what to do.

Modifying Human Behavior

There are two general ways by which we can influence the actions of others. One is to concentrate on altering their ideas, feelings, or goals; the other is to change the situation, thereby indirectly affecting their goals, ideas, and feelings. We often combine these approaches.

We strive for prevention of accidents through modification of human behavior through one or more of the following *modes of influence:*

1. By conveying new information (education).
2. By advising (effective according to the prestige of the source: his presumed experience, knowledge, and judgment).
3. By giving commands which carry authority.
4. By appealing to values and sentiments (other than those invoked by positions of authority).
5. By giving inducements (offering something valued in return for compliance).
6. By using coercion (threat of harm, the opposite of inducement; it can be a form of inducement: "If you do as I wish, then I won't do what you'd rather I'd not do").
7. By using force, with or without authority (the threat of force is coercion).

[6] David Rosenhan, Frank Frederick, and Anne Burrowes, "Preaching and Practicing Effects of Channel Discrepancy on Norm Internalization," *Child Development*, XXXIX (March, 1968), 291–301.

[7] William L. Carlson and David Klein, "Familial vs. Institutional Socialization of the Young Traffic Offender," *Journal of Safety Research*, II, No. 1 (March 1970), 13–25.

It should be noted that behavior modification usually begins with education and continues down through the influence of each successive mode if the preceding one is not effective.

Dr. William Haddon, Jr. gives some examples of the continuum of behavior modification in accident prevention:

> The prevention of accidents through the modification of human behavior is usually approached through (1) education, (2) coercion, and (3) legal sanctions. In general, when educational efforts have failed, coercion has been tried; when this has failed, legal sanctions have been endorsed. However, when neither education nor coercive measures have proved effective, the implementation of the last step has often taken decades. This was seen in the quarter-of-a-century lag between the development of the railroad air brake and automatic coupler and the passage of legislation that forced their general use—a period in which tens of thousands of railroad workers were killed and many more injured. This is also illustrated by the long lag between the required use of safety belts in aircraft and their mandatory installation in new automobiles and by the interval in the United States of some fifty years between the first public recognition that the drinking driver is a highway menace and the enactment of laws permitting his identification through the use of breath and other quantitative chemical tests.[8]

The bases of influence are numerous. We can include among the most important position in an organization (e.g., a command post in an army), money, social connections, prestige as a result of past performances, knowledge, skill, and physical characteristics (e.g., strength, height, sex appeal).

Some major factors which account for the long lag in applying acquired knowledge include the following:

1. New knowledge is emerging in greater profusion with more rapidity than ever before.
2. There are far too few trained personnel, facilities, and resources for us to make use of new knowledge.
3. Various public attitudes toward the accident problem inhibit prevention efforts (as we noted in Chapter 1).
4. Measures to reduce accident injury and death demand continuous individual effort.

Let us return now to objectives *1.–6.* and determine how well you have achieved them.

[8] William Haddon, Jr., "The Prevention of Accidents," in *Preventive Medicine,* eds. Duncan W. Clark and Brian MacMahon (Boston: Little, Brown, and Company, 1967), p. 598.

6 determinants affecting the safety movement

After reading this chapter, you should be able to:

1. *Name organizations, their major emphasis, and their contributions to safety.*
2. *Give examples of disasters and their influence upon accident reduction.*
3. *List technological developments and state reasons for resistance in their acceptance.*
4. *Appraise safety legislation.*
5. *Evaluate the influence of monetary costs in accident prevention.*

The Safety Trend [1]

Probably accidents have always plagued mankind. One of the earliest accounts of safety concern occurs in the eighth verse of the twenty-second chapter of Deuteronomy: "When thou buildest a new house, then thou shalt make a battlement for thy roof, that thou bring not blood upon thine house, if any man fall from thence." From this early admonition until the Industrial Revolution of the 1800's, accidents were the concern of the individual. The Industrial Revolution brought many changes—new hazards and new responsibilities which affected more people.

[1] Herbert J. Stack and J. Duke Elkow, *Education for Safe Living* (Englewood Cliffs, N.J.: Prentice-Hall, Inc., 1966). See Chapter One, for a detailed account of the history of the safety movement.

Factory inspections were introduced in England as early as 1833 and were designed to alleviate some of the worst hazards. But not until the twentieth century was any really effective attack made upon industrial hazards.[2] Governmental regulations and controls were gradually formulated by most states in this country.

The most effective labor legislation was passed between 1910 and 1915 and consisted of workmen's compensation laws. These laws required that the employer contribute to the costs of any work injury, whether or not a worker had been negligent.

Increased interest in safety also resulted in the formation of the National Safety Council in 1912. Initially formed out of concern for industrial safety, this agency was later expanded to include all aspects of safety and accident prevention.

We realize how effective the safety movement is by examining accident rates for the past several decades. In general, statistics available for work or industrial accidents indicate a definite decrease. However, trends over the years for motor-vehicle accidents have been less encouraging although mortality rates based on deaths per 10,000 motor vehicles and per 100,000,000 road miles have shown a decrease. Fatal home accidents show an unfavorable trend over the years—there has been little change in yearly totals. Thus death rates for household accidents have dropped because the total population has increased.

The accident problem remains a significant one. There is still much room for improvement.

The National Safety Council reports that from the formation of their council in 1912 to the present, accidental deaths per 100,000 population have decreased 30 percent, and if the rate had not decreased, nearly 1,500,000 more people would have died as a result of accidents.[3] Of course the success of death prevention is a result of efforts of many organizations and individuals to alleviate accidental death.

Organizations and Agencies

Consistent and organized safety efforts have reduced the toll of accidents that otherwise might have reached considerable proportions. Various organizations emphasized to varying degrees what is known as the "three E" concept for accident prevention: *E*ngineering, *E*nforcement, and *E*ducation. Table 6–1 lists some of these organizations which are

[2] H. W. Heinrich, *Industrial Accident Prevention* (New York: McGraw-Hill Book Company, 1931), p. 366.

[3] National Safety Council, *Accident Facts* (Chicago: National Safety Council, 1970), p. 10.

TABLE 6–1   **Organizations and Agencies**

ENGINEERING	ENFORCEMENT	EDUCATION
National Highway Traffic Safety Administration	National Highway Traffic Safety Administration	National Highway Traffic Safety Administration
University Safety Centers	University Safety Centers	University Safety Centers
National Safety Council	National Safety Council	National Safety Council
Highway User's Federation for Safety and Mobility	Highway User's Federation for Safety and Mobility	Highway User's Federation for Safety and Mobility
American Society of Safety Engineers	U.S. Coast Guard	American National Red Cross
National Board of Fire Underwriters	State and local law enforcement agencies	National Rifle Association
Underwriters' Laboratories, Inc.	American Association of Motor Vehicle Administrators	American Driver and Traffic Safety Association
	American Bar Association	American Association of Health, Physical Education, and Recreation
		American Automobile Association

concerned with various phases of the "three E" concept. The list is by no means exhaustive or comprehensive in identifying those agencies and organizations with a specific interest in safety.

The safety educator or specialist can keep well informed and abreast of current safety issues, by subscribing or referring to the periodicals suggested in Table 6–2.

Disasters

Chapter 3 briefly deals with the number of deaths resulting from disasters. As you will recall, the number of deaths from disasters is proportionately small when compared with other causes of accidental death; yet events called disasters receive front-page coverage in newspapers and news magazines.

The loss of life from disasters has decidedly influenced attempts to prevent needless death and injury. Table 6–3 presents a list of disasters with their respective death tolls and, more important, includes efforts made for reducing death and injury following these disasters.

TABLE 6–2   **Safety Periodicals**

NAME OF PERIODICAL	WHEN PUBLISHED	ADDRESS
Traffic Safety	Monthly	National Safety Council 425 North Michigan Ave. Chicago, Ill. 60611
Family Safety	Quarterly	''
School Safety	Bi-monthly	''
Farm Safety Review	Bi-monthly	''
National Safety News	Monthly	''
National Safety Congress Transactions	Annually	''
Journal of Safety Research	Quarterly	''
Behavioral Research in Highway Safety	Quarterly	Behavioral Publications 2852 Broadway-Morningside Heights New York, N.Y. 10025
Journal of the American Society of Safety Engineers	Monthly	American Society of Safety Engineers 850 Busse Highway Park Ridge, Ill. 60068
Journal of Traffic Safety Education	Bi-monthly except sum- mer months	California Driver Education Association 413 Dahlia Corona del Mar, Calif. 92625
Statistical Bulletin	Monthly	Metropolitan Life Insurance Co. One Madison Avenue New York, N.Y. 10010
Annual Safety Education Review	Annually	American Association of Health, Physical Education, and Recreation 1201 Sixth Street, N.W. Washington, D.C.
Traffic Digest and Review	Monthly	Traffic Institute Northwestern University 1804 Hinman Avenue Evanston, Ill. 60204
Analogy	Quarterly	Allstate Insurance Company Allstate Plaza Northbrook, Ill. 60062
Concepts	Quarterly	Aetna Life and Casualty 151 Farmington Avenue Hartford, Conn. 06115

The Galveston tidal wave of September 8, 1900, in which approximately 6,000 lives were lost, was the most devastating disaster on record in the United States. A cyclone and tidal wave on November 12, 1970, struck East Pakistan resulting in a disaster of proportions unprecedented in this

TABLE 6–3   **Disasters and Their Effects Upon Safety**

TYPE	LOCATION AND DATE	TOTAL DEATHS	RESULTS
Fire	City of Chicago, Illinois October 9, 1871	250	Building codes prohibiting wooden structures; water reserve
Flood	Johnstown, Pennsylvania May 31, 1889	2,209	Inspections
Tidal wave	Galveston, Texas September 8, 1900	6,000	Sea wall built
Fire	Iroquois Theatre, Chicago, Ill. December 30, 1903	575	Stricter theater safety standards
Marine	"General Slocum" burned; East River, New York June 15, 1904	1,021	Stricter ship inspections; revision of statutes (life preservers, experienced crew, fire extinguishers)
Earthquake and fire	San Francisco, California April 18, 1906	452	Widened streets, limited heights of buildings, steel frame and fire resistant buildings
Mine	Monogah, West Virginia December 6, 1907	361	Creation of Federal Bureau of Mines; stiffened mine inspections
Fire	North Collinwood School, Cleveland, Ohio March 8, 1908	176	Need realized for fire drills and planning of school structures
Fire	Triangle Shirt Waist Co., New York March 25, 1911	145	Strengthening of laws concerning alarm signals, sprinklers, fire escapes, fire drills
Marine	Titanic struck iceberg, Atlantic Ocean April 15, 1912	1,517	Regulation regarding number of lifeboats; all passenger ships equipped for around-the-clock radio watch; International Ice Patrol
Explosion	New London School, Texas March 18, 1937	294	Odorants put in natural gas
Fire	"Coconut Grove," Boston, Mass. November 28, 1942	492	Ordinances regulating aisle space, electrical wiring, flame-proofing of decorations, overcrowding, signs indicating the maximum number of occupants; administration of blood plasma to prevent shock and the use of penicillin
Plane	Two-plane air collision over Grand Canyon, Arizona June 30, 1956	128	Controlled airspace expanded, use of infrared as a warning indicator

Source: Based upon information from *Accident Facts* (1970), p. 21, by permission of the National Safety Council.

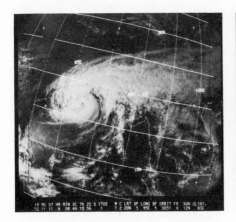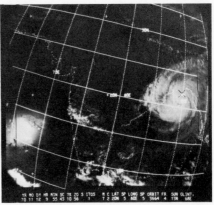

FIGURE 6–1 **This cyclone (hurricane) in the Bay of Bengal, 1970, produced the century's worst disaster. This photo was taken from an unmanned weather satellite, ITOS-1. Reproduced courtesy of the National Oceanic and Atmospheric Administration.**

century (see Fig. 6–1). The cost in lives from this natural disaster will never be reckoned accurately—a loss of more than half a million lives has been estimated. Most of you will well remember one or more of the major disasters which occurred in the United States as listed in Table 6–4.

The world's worst disaster on record (other than the Biblical account of Noah and the flood) occurred in A.D. 1887; a flood took 900,000 lives along the Hwang Ho River in China's Honan Province.

Technology

We become aware of the impact of technology on safety and accident loss reduction by looking at various innovations (see Fig. 6–2 a–d). Whether the innovation be safety lenses (eye glasses), safety belts (lap and harness types in automobiles), safety hats (steel or other hard material), safety shoes (steel-toed), or safety guards (on electrical saws)—all of which are widely accepted today—we can be sure that formerly they were viewed as quite unacceptable and met with widespread resistance. One prime obstacle to change is *habit*. Only when many people recognize a problem do we consider change and search about for new ways of doing things. Perhaps there are several reasons for the survival of many unsafe practices and technological methods: people are used to these practices and methods, people accept the fact that accidents will happen, and people hesitate to adopt new ways for preventing accidents because it involves effort.

TABLE 6–4 **Major Catastrophes in Order of Significance**
(*Accidents Taking 25 or More Lives, United States, 1965–1970*)

DATE	PLACE	TYPE OF ACCIDENT	NUMBER OF LIVES LOST
1970			
November 14	Huntington, W. Va.	Crash of chartered jetliner	75
December 30	Wooton, Ky.	Explosion in coal mine	38
January	Marietta, Ohio	Nursing home fire	31
October 2	Near Silver Plume, Colo.	Crash of chartered plane	31
December 20	Tucson, Ariz.	Hotel fire	28
May 11	Lubbock, Texas	Tornado	26
April 17–18	Texas Panhandle	Tornadoes	25
1969			
August 17	Mississippi and Louisiana	Hurricane	200
September 9	Near Indianapolis, Ind.	Collision of commercial airliner with private plane	83
August 20	Virginia	Floods in aftermath of hurricane	80
January 20–26	California	Rain, floods, and subsequent mud slides	43
July 4	Near Los Angeles, Calif.	Plunge of commercial airliner into Pacific	38
January 18	Southern Mississippi	Tornadoes	32
April 6	New Orleans, La.	Collision of oil barge and freighter	25
1968			
May 3	Near Dawson, Texas	Crash of commercial airliner	85
November 20	Near Mannington, W. Va.	Explosion and fire in coal mine	78
May 15	Midwest	Tornadoes	71
April 6	Richmond, Ind.	Explosion and fire in sporting goods shop	43
August 10	Charleston, W. Va.	Crash of commercial airliner	35
October 25	Near Hanover, N.H.	Crash of commercial airliner into mountain peak in fog	32
December 27	Chicago, Ill.	Collision of commercial airliner	28

1967

Date	Location	Event	Number
July 19	Near Hendersonville, N.C.	Collision of commercial airliner with private plane	82
November 20	Near Cincinnati, Ohio	Crash of commercial airliner near airport	70
April 21	Northeastern Illinois	Tornadoes	55
December 15	Near Pt. Pleasant, W. Va.	Collapse of bridge	46
March 5	Near Kenton, Ohio	Crash of commercial airliner in storm	38
July 16	Berrydale, Fla.	Prison camp barracks swept by fire	38
June 23	Near Blossburg, Pa.	Collision of commercial airliner	34
March 9	Near Urbana, Ohio	Collision of commercial airliner with private plane	26
February	Montgomery, Ala.	Penthouse restaurant swept by fire	25

1966

Date	Location	Event	Number
April 22	Near Ardmore, Okla.	Collision of military charter plane	83
March 3	Mississippi and Alabama	Tornadoes	58
August 6	Near Falls City, Neb.	Crash of commercial airliner in storm	42
June 16	Near Bayonne, N.J.	Collision of two tankers	33
March 22	Northern Great Plains	Blizzard	28
November 29	Near Harbor Beach, Mich.	Freighter sank in a Lake Huron storm	28

1965

Date	Location	Event	Number
April 11	Midwest	Tornadoes	272
September 8–10	South	Hurricane	88
February 8	Kennedy Int'l Airport, N.Y.	Plunge of commercial airliner into ocean	84
June 25	Near El Toro, Calif.	Crash of military plane into mountain	84
November 8	Near Cincinnati, Ohio	Crash of commercial airliner into hill	58
August 9	Near Searcy, Ark.	Explosion and fire at missile silo	53
November 11	Salt Lake City, Utah	Crash of commercial airliner	43
January 16	Wichita, Kansas	Crash of military plane into homes	30
August 16	Near Chicago, Ill.	Crash of commercial airliner into lake	30
June 18–19	Southwest	Floods	27

Source: Adapted from Metropolitan Life Insurance Company, *Statistical Bulletin*, January 1970 and February 1971, by permission of the Metropolitan Life Insurance Company.

51

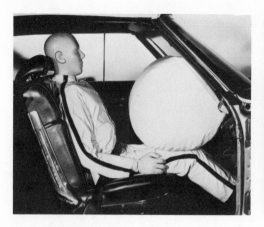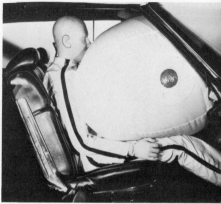

*FIGURE 6–2 a–d   **The automobile protective airbag—it may be the most
important safety development in recent years. Reproduced courtesy of the
National Highway Traffic Safety Administration and General Motors Cor-
poration.***

In addition to habit, *traditionalism* often lies behind some resistance to
innovation. Not only are people accustomed to present ways of doing
things, but they also revere these ways because people link them with the
past.

A third factor which leads to resistance to change is *vested interests.*
There are always groups of people in advantageous positions who would
feel their status threatened by change. Most of the issues in safety presented in Chapter 4 represent groups of people with vested interests.

Legislation

Usually laws are enacted as a "last resort" after other attempts to
control behavior have failed. Legislation also appears as an aftermath
of a disaster. A basic question that merits consideration is: "Can safety be
legislated?" There is little doubt that some regulatory legislation such as
that concerned with the design and operation of ships, trains, aircraft,
elevators, and mines, has contributed to the reduction of accident occurrence. We must do additional research, however, to determine the effectiveness of legislation. Nevertheless, the experience of one state dramatically
illustrates the effectiveness of safety legislation in saving lives. The state
of Michigan adopted a helmet requirement for motorcyclists in 1967, then
repealed it on the grounds of unconstitutionality in 1968. When motorcycle fatalities rose 42 percent that year, Michigan quickly reenacted the
statute.

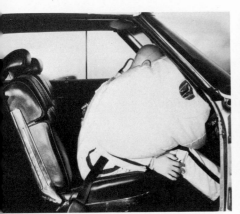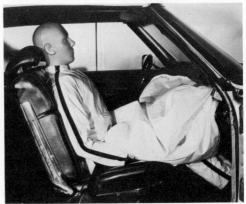

Regrettably, there are some who believe "laws are made to be broken" and "if you disagree with a law, it's all right to break it." Equally unfortunate, it appears that people have to be forced into safer behavior patterns.

Happily, there are a few outstanding examples of safety legislation: workmen's compensation acts, motor-vehicle codes, mine safety bills, toy safety regulations, consumer product safety acts, and various fire and building safety regulations.

Economic Costs

A very strong motivational factor is the gain or loss of money. Few people make money from accidents; if any do, someone else is losing it. Extremely large amounts of money have been lost in accident costs; these costs have provided strong impetus for accident prevention. "Touch a man's pocketbook and he becomes alarmed" is quite an accurate and relevant statement. In Chapter 3, we listed several economic consequences of accidents.

Let us return now to objectives *1.–5.* and determine how well you have achieved them.

7 safety instruction: an approach to accident prevention

After reading this chapter, you should be able to:

1. Differentiate between instruction, teaching, and education.
2. Identify the instructional model and define its four component parts.
3. Identify a behavioral objective which meets the three requirements stated by Robert F. Mager.
4. Point out the advantages of preassessing students.
5. Select appropriate learning activities which enable behavioral objectives to be achieved.
6. Point out what the results of evaluation indicate.
7. Plan a lesson which describes the things which will enable a student and/or class to reach expected outcomes.
8. Evaluate the use of "fear" in safety instruction.
9. Define "cognitive dissonance."
10. Give examples of the effectiveness of safety instruction in reducing accident occurrence.

Instruction Is Different

Instruction is a special kind of teaching with specific purposes and a systematic organization that is not characteristic of all teaching. Education and teaching and instruction are not interchangeable concepts as most people believe. The relationship of the three is pictured in Figure 7–1. Education is broad and all-encompassing, and includes all those experiences which enhance the individual's knowledge, whether through the formal classroom, television, or parental counsel. Teaching occurs most often in a classroom, but as most teachers readily admit, it includes extra-curricular activities as well. Instruction does not involve the complexity of teaching. It does not include such concerns as classroom management or discipline, collecting club dues, supervising recess periods, or a host of other skills which in most cases only on-the-job experience can provide. Of course, there are instances of good teaching and education for which the objectives cannot be defined and the instructional procedures are not predetermined. However, for several years in the United States there has been an encouraging emphasis upon better instruction. An outcome of this emphasis has been the development of behavioral objectives and systematic instruction. Developing lesson plans and courses based upon behavioral objectives and appropriate instructional activities will be the major criteria for revising most future curricula. Haberman indicates this

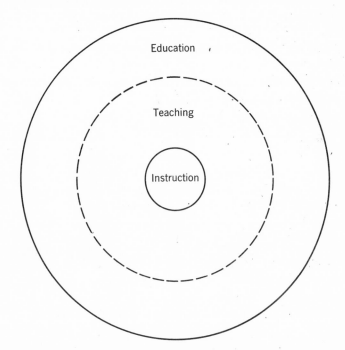

FIGURE 7–1 **Relation of instruction, teaching, and education. *Adapted from Phil C. Lange, ed., "Introduction," in* Programmed Instruction, The Sixty-sixth Yearbook of the National Society for the Study of Education (Chicago: The University of Chicago Press, 1967), p. 4, by permission of the NSSE.**

when he states: "They cannot be ignored and must be contended with, since this approach promises to be the major vehicle for revising curriculum in the future." [1]

Instructional Model

There is no single concept, theory, or method of teaching or instruction, and probably never will be. For example, the Socratic method of teaching stresses inquiry, dialectic (conversation between the teacher and the student), and inductive logic. Those who follow the Jesuit method of education are described as "masters of method"; they emphasize rote learning. Yet both of these approaches and others have been successful to varying degrees.

One of the most recent and useful emphases in education is what is known as a "systematic approach" to instruction. We may compare this "systematic approach" to the vacationing tourist who travels with a predetermined route marked on a road map. It is recognized that some good teachers may not adhere to the following ideas. However, their success was not the result of accidental or "off the cuff" inspiration, but rather the result of being well organized, informed, inventive, and skillful in presenting their concepts to students.

This chapter is designed specifically with a framework to help you become a better safety instructor. Schaplowsky of the U.S. Public Health Service says that:

> [A]ccidents can be prevented by bringing about changes in man's environment and in his behavior. We know that behavior may be changed as a result of an increase in man's knowledge, improvement in his skills or modification of his attitudes.[2]

Schaplowsky continues by citing examples of traffic and scuba diving accidents, child poisonings, effects of carbon monoxide, and the dangers of ultra-thin plastic bags to illustrate the point that many accidents are the consequences of an individual's lack of knowledge. However, successful communication of factual knowledge does not necessarily guarantee successful modification of behavior. This applies to safety, algebra, English, and a myriad of subjects.

The lack of professional qualifications of safety instructors has been

[1] Martin Haberman, "Behavioral Objectives: Bandwagon or Breakthrough," *Journal of Teacher Education*, XIX (Spring 1963), 94.

[2] A. F. Schaplowsky, "What You Don't Know Can Hurt You," *School and College Safety*, National Safety Congress Transactions (Chicago: National Safety Council, 1961), 17.

implicated as one of the problems which results in their occasional ineffectiveness in influencing safe behavior. That the safety instructor must be highly qualified is well illustrated by Dr. Elkow:

> The New York Times editorialized last week on a shocking fact: "[H]alf the operations performed in American hospitals are done by physicians unqualified to perform in accordance with the standards of the American College of Surgeons." Equally shocking is the fact that safety education functions are carried on by persons *who,* at the time of their initial appointment or in some instances individuals currently functioning or about to function, are unqualified to meet the vital functions of preparing youth for safe living in our complex environment.[3]

Courses have been systematically developed for two areas of safety instruction. A project devised for the American Telephone and Telegraph Company by the American Institutes for Research had as its objective "to develop a basic first aid course which would, in seven and one-half hours, produce results at least equivalent to those produced by standard first aid instruction taking ten hours." Another instructional guide based upon behavioral objectives is *A Resource Curriculum in Driver and Traffic Safety Education* of the Highway Users Federation for Safety and Mobility, Washington, D.C.

The instructional model advocated in this chapter features four component parts or four essentially distinct operations. The definitions of the four parts are presented here; later sections of the chapter will be devoted to detailed consideration of each component part. Figure 7–2 depicts a flow chart which illustrates the sequential relationship of the four component parts of the instructional model. *Behavioral objectives* (box *A*) are the goals the student should attain upon completion of a segment of instruction. *Preassessment* (box *B*) is a determination of the student's current status with respect to the behavioral objectives. *Instruction* (box *C*) describes the activities that should bring about the intended student accomplishment as stated in the behavioral objectives. *Evaluation*

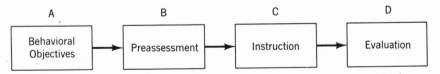

FIGURE 7–2   *The instructional model. Adapted from W. James Popham and Eva L. Baker, Systematic Instruction (Englewood Cliffs, N.J.: Prentice-Hall, Inc., 1970), p. 13, by permission of the publisher.*

[3] J. Duke Elkow, "College and University Advanced Courses in Safety Education," *School and College Safety,* National Safety Congress Transactions (Chicago: National Safety Council, 1961), p. 52.

(box *D*) consists of a means of determining how well the student has achieved the behavioral objectives. If the evaluation indicates that the student has fallen short of the standard of achievement (as stated in the behavioral objectives), an adjustment may be required in one of the essential parts of the instructional model, usually in the instructional component.[4]

Behavioral Objectives

Most instruction plans usually lack clear expression of behavioral objectives. Although most educators believe in objectives, past objectives or goals were based upon what the teacher had to accomplish or ambiguously described what the student was expected to achieve. Behavioral objectives describe explicitly how the student is expected to behave at the conclusion of instruction.

Robert F. Mager recommends that behavioral objectives include the following three parts:

1. Identification of the terminal performance or behavior which the instruction attempts to encourage. The verb in the statement of the objective identifies and names the action expected to be observed in the student.
2. Description of the important conditions under which the behavior is to occur. These conditions might include writing an examination, speaking orally in class, driving on a canyon road, or performing a particular skill on the job.
3. Description of the acceptable level of student performance. (Note that the behavioral objectives listed at the chapter beginnings of this textbook lack parts two and three.) Instructors might establish 90 percent correct answers on the examination, pass-or-fail performance of a job with safety checks, or consistently wear safety goggles while using a grinding machine as standards or expected levels of student performance.[5]

In insisting that the words chosen to state objectives (verbs depicting observable behavior) must not be open to misinterpretation, Mager supplies examples for consideration: [6]

---

[4] W. James Popham and Eva L. Baker, *Systematic Instruction* (Englewood Cliffs, N.J.: Prentice-Hall, Inc., 1970), p. 13.

[5] Adapted from Robert F. Mager, *Preparing Instructional Objectives* (Palo Alto, Calif.: Fearon Publishers, 1962), p. 53, by permission of the publisher.

[6] *Ibid.*, p. 11.

Words Open to Many Interpretations:

to know	to appreciate	to enjoy
to understand	to fully appreciate	to believe
to *really* understand	to grasp the significance of	to have faith in

Words Open to Fewer Interpretations:

to write	to differentiate	to list
to recite	to solve	to compare
to identify	to construct	to contrast

Examples of a variety of behavioral objectives are presented below. Notice that each states what the student will be doing as he demonstrates that he has achieved the stated objective; each also says something about the level of acceptable performance and under what conditions it should be reached. The form varies but this is not important; what is important is that expected student outcomes are made clear.

EXAMPLE 1

Using a copy of *Accident Facts,* the student should be able to classify ten home accidents as one of the eight types of home accidents.

EXAMPLE 2

As part of the final examination, the student should be able to list three disasters which took more than 25 lives in the United States last year.

EXAMPLE 3

Goal: Be able to point out community safety hazards.
Behavior: Identify dangerous conditions.
Conditions: The student will survey the community determined by the instructor.
Standards: Ten danger conditions.

EXAMPLE 4

Goal: Be familiar with terms commonly used in safety.
Behavior: Match term with correct definition.
Conditions: Given a list of terms and definitions.
Criterion: 8 correct matches out of 10.

There are different levels of behavior objectives such as lowest cognitive (rote memory or recall), higher-than-lowest cognitive (application, analysis, synthesis, evaluation, etc.), psychomotor (skills), and affective (attitude) levels. You might refer to the writings of Benjamin S. Bloom, Robert Gagne, W. James Popham, and M. David Merrill for further information and elaboration concerning different types or levels of behavioral objectives.

Preassessment

Preassessment is the process used to determine a student's level of attainment in relation to prescribed behavioral objectives. A teacher preassesses a student in two ways: (1) by knowing the student well enough to estimate his knowledge and background for the lesson before the class meets (evaluation at the conclusion of one lesson often aids in effective preassessment for a following lesson), and (2) by determining before or during the class period the student's knowledge of the lesson material and his ability to reach the behavioral objectives through, for example, his response to written diagnostic tests, oral questions, and general discussion. Instructors who preassess their students and instruct accordingly will probably avoid boring students with material already known and frustrating them with advanced material for which students lack the necessary background.

Instruction

Instruction consists of those activities in which a student engages to help him attain a behavioral objective. Notice that here we place emphasis on those things which a *student* does. Instructors use various methods and techniques which allow the student active participation in reaching the desired behavioral objectives.

There are many instructional methods and techniques. We may differentiate between a method and a technique by suggesting that a technique is a subtype of a method. For example, discussion is a method, whereas the specific types of discussion—question–answer, brainstorming, buzz groups, etc.—are techniques. An accurate guide which tells the instructor the best method or technique is nonexistent. In this section we will present some guidelines for the instructor's use in selecting appropriate instructional activities for his lesson.

Mager suggests that the selection of instructional procedures be based upon:

1. Choosing the technique which has conditions called for by the objective. If the objective calls for the student to analyze accident causes from newspaper accounts, then guided practice with newspaper accounts would be in order.

2. Choosing the technique which causes the student to perform in a manner called for by the objective. If the objective calls for the student to recognize potential community safety hazards, then guided observation through slides, a film, or a field trip to a segment of the community would be appropriate for practice in identifying potential hazards.[7]

Other considerations important to the proper selection of instructional activities are the grouping of students and the use of audio-visual aids. Table 7–1 shows us three kinds of classroom groupings and suggests activities for each. Note that some instructional activities may be utilized in one or more of the groups. In Tables 7–2 and 7–3 William H. Allen presents some factors for our consideration when using educational media or audio-visual aids as part of instructional activities.

In a later section you will find ideas and a suggested sequence for developing and unifying behavioral objectives, content, and instructional activities.

Evaluation

Evaluation is the process of comparing a student's behavior with the predetermined behavioral objective. Most often evaluation occurs in the final lesson or at the end of a lesson, although we may evaluate through a try-out experience during the lesson or in any applicable way. Evaluation may even take place during out-of-class periods in the form of an assignment.

The development of an evaluation procedure should derive specifically from the condition statement of the behavioral objective. Objectives and

TABLE 7–1 **Grouping for Instruction**

A. TEACHER ALONE	B. INTERACTION (between teacher and students or between students)	C. STUDENT ALONE
1. *lecture*	1. *buzz groups*	1. *reading*
2. *films*	2. *brainstorming*	2. *research*
3. *slides*	3. *question-answer discussion*	3. *programmed instruction*
4. *television*		4. *practice*
5. *guest speaker*	4. *committee work*	5. *writing*
6. *chalkboard*	5. *debates*	
7. *demonstration*	6. *role-playing*	

[7] Adapted from Robert F. Mager and Kenneth M. Beach, Jr., *Developing Vocational Instruction* (Palo Alto, Calif.: Fearon Publishers, 1967), p. 55, by permisssion of the publisher.

TABLE 7-2   *Relationship of Instructional Media Stimulus to Learning Objectives*

LEARNING OBJECTIVES

INSTRUCTIONAL MEDIA TYPE	LEARNING FACTUAL INFORMATION	LEARNING VISUAL IDENTIFICATIONS	LEARNING PRINCIPLES, CONCEPTS, AND RULES	LEARNING PROCEDURES	PERFORMING SKILLED PERCEPTUAL-MOTOR ACTS	DEVELOPING DESIRABLE ATTITUDES, OPINIONS, AND MOTIVATIONS
Still pictures	Medium	High	Medium	Medium	Low	Low
Motion pictures	Medium	High	High	High	Medium	Medium
Television	Medium	Medium	High	Medium	Low	Medium
3-D objects	Low	High	Low	Low	Low	Low
Audio recordings	Medium	Low	Low	Medium	Low	Medium
Programmed instruction	Medium	Medium	Medium	High	Low	Medium
Demonstration	Low	Medium	Low	High	Medium	Medium
Printed textbooks	Medium	Low	Medium	Medium	Low	Medium
Oral presentation	Medium	Low	Medium	Medium	Low	Medium

Source: Reprinted from William H. Allen, National Art Education Association government project report, which also appeared in "Media Stimulus and Types of Learning," *Audiovisual Instruction* (January 1967), p. 28, by permission of Association for Educational Communications & Technology.

TABLE 7–3   **Equipment/Media Relationships and Considerations**

INSTRUMENT	MEDIA USED	MATERIALS PRODUCTION CONSIDERATION	AVAILABILITY OF FACILITIES AND EQUIPMENT	EQUIPMENT COST
Filmstrip or slide projector	35mm. filmstrips or 2 × 2 slides	Inexpensive. May be done locally in short time.	Usually available. Requires darkened room	Low
Overhead transparency projector	Still pictures and graphic representations	Very inexpensive. May be done locally in short time.	Available. May be projected in light room.	Low
Wall charts or posters	Still pictures	Very inexpensive. May be done locally in a very short time.	Available. No special equipment needed.	Low
Motion pictures (projection to groups)	16mm. motion picture (sound or silent)	Specially-produced. Sound film is costly and requires 6–12 months time.	Usually available. Requires darkened classroom.	Moderate
Motion picture projection as repetitive loops (8mm. silent) to individuals	8mm. motion picture film (silent)	Special production normally necessary. May be produced as 16mm. film alone or locally at low cost and in very short time.	Not normally available. Will need to be specially procured to meet requirement of instructional program.	Low per unit, but moderate for groups.
Magnetic tape recorder	$\frac{1}{4}$" magnetic tape	Easy and inexpensive. Usually produced locally.	Available.	Low
Record player	33⅓, 45, or 78 rpm. disk recordings	Need special recording facilities. Usually commercially made.	Usually available.	Low
Display area	3-D models	May vary in complexity and in difficulty of production. Component parts easy to obtain.	Available.	Varies from low to high.
Television (closed circuit)	Live presentations. Motion picture film. Videotape recordings. Still pictures	Normally requires large and skilled production staff.	Not normally available.	Moderate to high.
Teaching machines and programmed textbooks	Programmed material	Some programs available commercially, but will normally be specially prepared for course.	Not normally available.	Low per unit, but moderate for groups.
System combinations	Television. Motion pictures. Still pictures. Audio recordings	Complex. Probably will be done locally to meet specific requirements.	Not normally available.	Moderate to high.

Source: Reprinted from William H. Allen National Art Education Association government project report, which also appeared in "Media Stimulus and Types of Learning," *Audiovisual Instruction* (January 1967), p. 31, by permission of the Association for Educational Communications & Technology.

evaluation should, in essence, be identical; that is, examination items should be drawn from the behavior specified in the objective to test for it. The following examples indicate objectives and appropriate evaluation:

EXAMPLE 1

Objective:
   On a written examination, the student will classify fires and indicate which type of fire extinguisher to use with 90 percent accuracy.
Evaluation:
   A list of fires (wood, gasoline, electrical, etc.) is given to the student. He identifies the fire class (A,B,C) to which each fire belongs and then indicates the best fire extinguisher (carbon dioxide, water, dry chemical, etc.) for each fire listed.

EXAMPLE 2

Objective:
   The student will safely control the steering of an automobile when a tire blows out or the air pressure suddenly diminishes.
Evaluation:
   While driving, a flat tire (blowout) simulator will release the air from a normal tire. The student will react effectively to this emergency situation by:
   (1) Firmly gripping the steering wheel and steering a straight course.
   (2) Easing up on the accelerator.
   (3) Braking with a firm and steady pressure (avoid "locking" wheels).
   (4) Looking for an escape route and driving entirely off the roadway.
   (5) Securing the car (putting parking brake and selector lever in park).

This prevents the use of tests that are really "guessing games," which often occurs in our schools. If one follows this procedure and students then fail to attain the predescribed goals, the instructor may be responsible; either his plans have been inadequate or he has not carried them out well. However, if the behavioral objectives are achieved, the instructor deserves much credit. When this instructional procedure is followed successfully, norm-referenced or curve grading (which guarantees a definite number of successes and failures) becomes archaic.

Lesson Plans

The lesson plan is the instructional blueprint that describes those activities which will enable the student or class to reach that lesson's behavioral objectives. Some teachers are admonished for following a lesson plan but such plans are important. However, there are probably as many different formats for lesson plans as there are instructors: what works well for one instructor may not work so well for another. Most important, the instructor must feel comfortable with his lesson plan.

The lesson plan format in Table 7–4 is a suggested one. The suggested plan does not apply to psychomotor (skill) lessons. This plan consists of: behavioral objectives, concepts or ideas to be taught for each behavioral objective, appropriate learning activities, and appropriate evaluation for the behavioral objectives. The ideas to be presented form the content outline.

Table 7–5 depicts a sequence of learning activities entitled *show, discuss,* and *apply* and suggests activities for each. The "cone of experience" shown in Table 7–6 provides additional aid by helping the instructor to determine which experiences or activities will be most effective

TABLE 7–4   **Sample Lesson Plan Form**

Title: _____

Objectives:

   1.

   2.

Materials needed:

Preassessment:

Ideas To Be Taught	Learning Activities
1.	Show:
	Discuss:
	Apply:
2.	Show:
	Discuss:
	Apply:

Evaluation:

  In class:

  Following class:

Assignment:

TABLE 7–5   **Learning Activities**

SHOW *	DISCUSS	APPLY
Show the class what you want them to learn through use of:	*Engage the class in discussion to:*	*Encourage the application of ideas and concepts through:*
Objects	*Raise questions*	*Assignments*
Pictures	*Cite and elicit examples*	*In-class activities which re-*
Stories	*Pose problems*	*quire students to use ideas*
Charts	*Consider various points*	*Specific out-of-class projects*
Diagrams	*of view*	*which challenge students*
Films	*Seek reasons*	*Follow-up measures to en-*
Real experiences		*sure good results*
(past and present)		
Recordings		
Role playing		
Textbook content		

* This step should serve as an effective interest-arouser and provide a common background experience which can be used later as a reference point for discussion. It is most effective when it is stimulating and eye-catching although reference to a previous group experience can also be very effective.

Source: Adapted from Asahel D. Woodruff, *Basic Concepts of Teaching* (San Francisco: Chandler Publishing Company, 1961), pp. 93ff.

for *show*. Specific examples of activities for each segment of the "cone of experience" are found in Table 7–7.

Sample completed lesson plans are provided to aid the reader to conceptualize better the ideas of this section (Tables 7–8 and 7–9).

The "Scare" Technique

The scare technique has been employed in safety education for many years. A fear or scare can shake people out of indifference and apathy toward productive change, and sometimes the use of shock techniques seems justified and necessary. However, in safety education, the use of fear to change attitudes can backfire because fear that generates apprehension can be destructive.

Researchers have come to the following conclusions regarding the use of scare techniques to change or influence behavior:

1. Fear methods tend to be short-term in their effectiveness.
2. Fear techniques can influence behavior by leading to constructive change or by preventing one from doing something dangerous. Strong fear techniques have been reported to produce no change in behavior whereas minimal fear techniques have been more

TABLE 7–6   The Cone of Learning Experiences

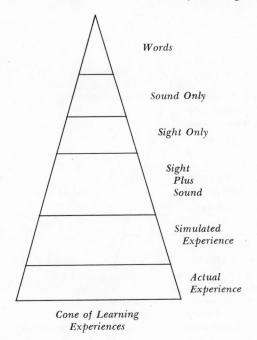

Words

Sound Only

Sight Only

Sight
Plus
Sound

Simulated
Experience

Actual
Experience

*Cone of Learning
Experiences*

The cone suggests that:

A. *Certain experiences are closer to or further from direct experience.*

B. *When we use more than one of our senses our learning is more complete. Usually the closer we get to the bottom of the cone the more senses we use.*

The cone provides knowledge which enables us to decide the appropriate learning experience to use after we consider the following interrelated factors:

A. *The readiness of the students in terms of their experiences with something.*

B. *The cost of the experience in terms of money, effort, time or safety.*

Often the best instructional decision involves use of learning activities in the lower area of the cone. ⟶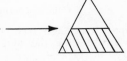

However, the decision to use activities in the upper area of the cone may be appropriate when the two factors above are considered. ⟶

Source: Adapted from Edgar Dale, *Audio-Visual Methods in Teaching.* Copyright © 1969 by The Dryden Press, Inc., by permission of The Dryden Press, Inc., and Baird, et al., *A Behavioral Introduction to Teaching* (Dubuque, Iowa: Kendall & Hunt, 1970), p. 90, by permission of the authors.

TABLE 7–7   *Cone of Experience Worksheet*

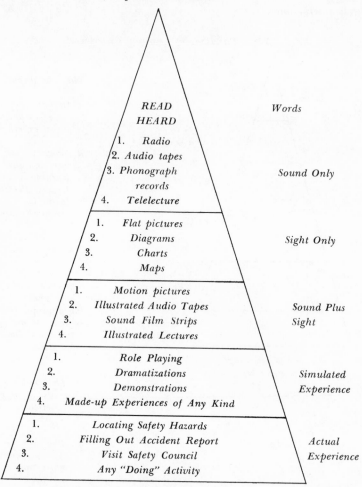

READ

HEARD

Words

1. Radio
2. Audio tapes
3. Phonograph
   records
4. Telelecture

Sound Only

1. Flat pictures
2. Diagrams
3. Charts
4. Maps

Sight Only

1. Motion pictures
2. Illustrated Audio Tapes
3. Sound Film Strips
4. Illustrated Lectures

Sound Plus
Sight

1. Role Playing
2. Dramatizations
3. Demonstrations
4. Made-up Experiences of Any Kind

Simulated
Experience

1. Locating Safety Hazards
2. Filling Out Accident Report
3. Visit Safety Council
4. Any "Doing" Activity

Actual
Experience

Cone of Learning Experiences

Source: Adapted from Edgar Dale, *Audio-Visual Methods in Teaching.* Copyright ©
1969 by The Dryden Press, Inc., by permission of The Dryden Press, Inc.

successful. Yet it has been reported that those with little experience with the subject matter react favorably after a strong fear
appeal. Divergent opinions exist among researchers.

3. Fear techniques can adversely affect some people by causing
   worry and anxiety.
4. Fear is a learned response.
5. If fear techniques are used too often, a person may become
   "calloused" or too accustomed to their use for any desired behavior change to occur.
6. There is need for further research—there is no single answer
   regarding the effectiveness of scare techniques. Few studies on

TABLE 7–8   **Sample Lesson Plan**

Title:
Multiple-Cause Concept of Accident Causation

Objective:
After completion of this lesson each class member should be able to define the multiple-cause concept, and identify the implications this concept has for safe behavior.

Materials needed:
1. *16 mm. film projector.*
2. *Film: "The Final Factor" color, 14 minutes, 1968, purchase or lease from AAA Foundation for Traffic Safety.*
3. *Copies of a newspaper accident account for each student (double spaced with wide margins).*

Preassessment:
Some class members may be well-acquainted with the multiple-cause concept. Ask who is and have them assist you during the lesson by giving illustrations of factors from their accident experiences to portray the multiple-cause concept.

CONCEPT OR IDEA TO BE TAUGHT	LEARNING ACTIVITIES
Accidents generally result from a combination of human-agent-environmental factors acting in a closely interwoven fashion (multiple-cause concept).	*Show:* Show the film "The Final Factor."
	Discuss: Ask: *What is the main concept or idea in the film?*
	Ask: *What are the implications for safe behavior?*
	Ask: *Does the multiple-cause concept apply to all accidents?*
	Ask: *Does anyone know of an accident for which several known influential factors existed?*
	Apply: Hand out a newspaper account of an accident to each student. Have students circle words, phrases, and/or sentences which might describe factors of accident causation. Write marginal notes if appropriate.

Evaluation:
In class: The newspaper exercise could be used.

Following class: During the week read the newspaper. Choose one account of an accident and circle the key words, phrases, and/or sentences which might indicate factors affecting the accident. Write marginal notes if appropriate. Turn the article in next week.

Assignment:
Read sections in the textbook appropriate for the next topic of class consideration.

TABLE 7-9   *Sample Lesson Plan*

Title:
Emergency First Aid at an Accident Scene

Objective:
The student should be able to identify recommended first-aid procedures for accident cases.

Materials needed:
Situation described below typed and duplicated for each class member.

Preassessment:
Ask for volunteers to demonstrate the systematic examination of a victim for injuries and life-threatening problems.

CONCEPT OR IDEA TO BE TAUGHT	LEARNING ACTIVITIES
When accidents occur, it is essential that every effort be made to save lives and lessen the severity of injuries. Good first aid training is essential	Show: Hand out copies of the accident situation. Read it to the class or have students read it.

Situation

You are the first to arrive at the scene of a two-car collision. Both cars are up-right. A quick survey of the scene reveals the following victims:

Car 1: The driver is unconscious and seated in the front seat fastened by his safety belt. The head of the passenger in the front seat has been thrown through the windshield. He is bleeding profusely about the face, is unconscious, with shallow respiration.

Car 2: The driver is seated in the front seat. He is sweating and appears to be short of breath. He complains of severe pain in his chest and left arm. The passenger has been thrown from the car. He is lying on the road moaning that he cannot move his legs. He appears to feel no sensation in his legs.

Discuss:
1. What is most likely wrong with each victim?
2. Which victim should be treated first and why?
3. What care should be given to each victim?
4. Which victim should be transported first and why?

Evaluation:
In class: Hand out another typed description of a first-aid accident situation to which students may respond individually (similar to an examination).

Following class: Prepare one accident situation (actual case, if possible) and respond to it by indicating the appropriate first aid measures to be taken.

Assignment:
Read all assigned material to date in preparation for the final examination.

70

use of fear techniques exist specifically in safety education. It is advised that until more evidence is shown that the safety educator use fear sparingly.

Cognitive Dissonance

Generally, people are consistent in their behavior; however, there is an inconsistency sometimes between what a person knows and the behavior pattern he chooses to follow. We call this *cognitive dissonance.* For example, many people believe that the driver of an automobile should wear a safety belt but a sizable number of people who believe this do not actually fasten safety belts (70 percent according to the National Safety Council [8]). Thus, dissonance exists between their beliefs and their behavior.[9]

Safety Instruction Effectiveness

Evidence to date indicates that safety instruction can be effective. For example, the Utah Fish and Game Department has shown through its mandatory gun-safety training program that firearm accidents can be dramatically reduced. Statistics for 1957 when the program was inaugurated, show that of 165,081 hunters who went afield, 22 were fatally injured. As the program gained momentum, the number of deaths among hunters dropped to twelve in 1959, to seven in 1960, and to five in 1961. Since 1961, the number has fluctuated between four and eight per year. The total number of fatal and nonfatal hunting accidents plummeted from 126 in 1957 to about an annual rate of 20 in recent years. The incidence of juvenile hunting accidents dropped even more spectacularly, plunging from 93 annually to as few as three or four per year. During the same period, the number of licensed adult hunters doubled and the number of juvenile nimrods increased fivefold.

Driver education in American high schools is presently our most popular, most widely applied, and probably most expensive safety instructional program. This course usually consists of both classroom and laboratory phases. In recent years, most United States public high schools provide such a course to youth approaching the legal driving age.

One criticism of high school driver education courses is that there is

8 National Safety Council, *Accident Facts* (Chicago: National Safety Council, 1970), 53.

9 See Leon Festinger, *The Theory of Cognitive Dissonance* (Evanston, Ill.: Row and Peterson, 1957), for more information.

no research evidence in terms of accident and driving violation records to prove the value of the course. Dozens of studies have been made which generally support driver education programs.

A report of the *Secretary's Advisory Committee on Traffic Safety* to the U.S. Department of Health, Education and Welfare (known as the "Moynihan Report") was presented by the press as representing an anti-driver education position. One statement from this report bears repeating and offers a rebuttal to those who oppose driver education:

> Now, at the hopeful beginnings of a new era, it becomes necessary to give a new cast to driver education. Although there is no conclusive proof as to the comparative effectiveness of various driver education techniques or, for that matter, the whole of present driver education practice, there is even less proof of the efficacy and value of any alternatives to present practices for communicating to the young person the rudiments of how to handle a car in modern traffic, and the associated social responsibilities. But operational driver education programs must continue. The problem is no different in principle than that for education in general. We have to continue with present systems even while recognized needed improvements are being studied. One would hardly advocate a moratorium on all schooling while looking for proof of better methods.[10]

We now find many who say that the emphasis should be diverted from educational efforts concerned with averting accidents to those efforts which assume accidents will occur and place emphasis on prevention of further loss through the widespread use of passive restraint systems (air bag in automobiles), collapsible steering wheels, and other innovations. Use of these devices will certainly reduce the number of deaths and critical injuries sustained in motor-vehicle crashes.

Walter Kohl offers another very discerning suggestion with regard to the placement of emphasis by saying that:

> Building more reliable devices, safer cars, better highways, is all to the good, but as one observer said, "it is similar to the attempt of reducing the occurrence of crime by making it harder to steal, or to kill, rather than by improving the social climate." The attitude of people is the basic issue. This attitude cannot be managed, but only improved slowly by the individual's acceptance of a different set of values.[11]

It would seem that through educational efforts we can truly affect attitudes. The critics of safety education programs do not intend to

[10] U.S. Department of Health, Education and Welfare, *Report to the Secretary's Advisory Committee on Traffic Safety* (Washington, D.C.: U.S. Government Printing Office, 1968), p. 63.

[11] Walter H. Kohl, "Can Accidents Be Managed?" *Journal of the American Society of Safety Engineers*, XIII, No. 11 (November 1968), 12.

eliminate safety courses, but believe these programs should rely on scientific evaluation for their justification rather than mere "common sense." Any safety educator should want the same.

Let us return now to objectives *1.–10.* and determine how well you have achieved them.

8 *readings*

When Is an Accident Not an Accident?

JOHN J. BROWNFAIN

The common definition and fatalistic connotation of the word "accident" appears to be an obstacle to accident prevention efforts. Few events labeled accidents really are accidents in the sense that they are purely chance events. Accidents are caused and, therefore, can be controlled when their causes are identified and understood. Resultant accident loss is a consequence of an unplanned event and does not in itself constitute the accident. Thus this article explores the most common word in safety—"accident."

It is interesting and instructive to contrast the way we use the word "accident" in everyday life and in the field of psychology. Ordinarily, we mean by "accident" some undesired or unintended event has taken place resulting in damage to persons or to property. On the other hand, in psychology an accident is an event caused by factors which are outside of the system to which the event belongs. Once the cause of an event becomes known and understood, the effect can no longer be called an accident.

It is the task of psychology and of other sciences to refine and expand its theoretical systems and models so that ultimately all events in the system can be understood, predicted, and controlled. The closer science comes to this ideal the more successful it is in eliminating or reducing accidents.

The difference between these two meanings of accident is truly fundamental and it is worth reflecting about. In our everyday usage, we resort to the word accident not merely to describe a misfortune, but also to offer

Reprinted from John J. Brownfain, "When Is an Accident Not an Accident?" *Journal of the American Society of Safety Engineers* (September 1962), pp. 19–20, by permission of the American Society of Safety Engineers. Copyright © 1962 by the American Society of Safety Engineers.

our apology in advance. In essence we are saying that something unpleasant or even calamitous has happened, but we are not to be blamed.
It is not our fault because it was an accident. It was inevitable and it
would have happened to anyone. Thus we remove ourselves from personal
responsibility.

Note, however, that this common usage of accident refers to the unfortunate outcome of an event and not to the cause. To someone examining the system and taking the scientific point of view, the not to be wished
for outcome might be highly predictable and not an accident at all. We
even refer to unwanted babies as accidents. But anyone who is enough
of a scientist to know what goes into the making of babies would surely
agree that the result is highly predictable.

Not Accident if Cause Is Known

All of which is to say that in science if you know the cause of an event,
that event is not an accident. In everyday life, on the other hand, if we
do not like the end result of this event and at the same time want to
escape personal responsibility for it, we are inclined to call it an accident.
Consider such components in a system as a group of teenagers, a beer
party, a car. Or such components as an adolescent and a shotgun assumed
to be unloaded, or a toddler and an open medicine chest, within easy
reach. These are the commonplace tragedies we read about every day.
Surely they are predictable, as predictable as the results of Russian roulette;
and, from the scientific point of view, not to be explained away as
accidents.

Roughly speaking, we can understand accidents as failures of systems
or of persons. Of course, a proper system needs to take account of persons
so that all accidents are failures in systems. However, to simplify our
analysis, it is still a good idea to take a separate look at persons and at
systems. To illustrate our point, let us first of all look at an accident
stemming from a defect in system. Recently in Binghamton, N.Y., a tragic
error occurred which resulted in the death of at least seven infants. We
do not have all the details, but it does appear that sugar and salt—which
are identical in appearance—were kept in containers located on the same
shelf, or at least in the same room. Salt was used in place of sugar in
preparing the infants' formula and a terrible disaster ensued.

Failure to Develop System

This was a consequence of a failure to develop a proper system. In a
sense, what took place was predictable and, while it was a tragedy, was

not strictly speaking an accident, if we are guided by our scientific definition. We can even formulate a law to the effect that a certain percentage
of the time when sugar and salt are in similar containers in the same area
they will be confused. Of course, there was human failure here too, but the
failure of the system stands out.

I have read that the system in Detroit hospitals is such that this particular accident could not have occurred. Now let us look at a celebrated
accident in Detroit which illustrates the failure of persons. I have in mind
the tragedy of the Great Wallendas. We are given to understand that the
key man in the pyramid was both inexperienced and ill—as it turned out,
a fatal combination. He refused to admit his illness, probably for the
reason that, in the interest of pride, he had to appear successful and
could not own up to his inadequacy no matter how temporary. Under
certain conditions, this might be an admirable trait, but in this instance
we must see it as the failure of a person.

Psychologists are interested both in failures of systems and of persons.
Many psychologists work in the field of engineering psychology. They are
interested in system development, and in fitting people to machines and
machines to people. Clinical psychologists like myself are more interested
in persons and in their failures. Obviously, both approaches are necessary
to do the total job. I know more about the failure of persons, and I would
like to offer a few remarks about this.

If you could find the perfect man and fit him into the perfect system,
there would be no accidents. This is an ideal, and while it might be
possible theoretically, it is not possible in an imperfect world. Let us
suppose you have an adequate system; the first thing you must do is to
select a man to attend to the system. This selection does not look for the
perfect man, but the right man. He must not be too little or too much
of anything. He mustn't be too dull for the job, and he mustn't be too
smart.

He must be devoted to duty, but not so devoted that he insists upon
reporting to work when he is sick and ought to be in bed. He ought to be
physically healthy in the way the system requires, but this need not
eliminate the physically handicapped. He ought to be emotionally healthy,
although we need not expect him to be entirely mature.

Emotional health is more difficult to evaluate than physical health,
but there are several indicators which are useful. We would want to
consider the stability of his work record, freedom from illness and accidents, and the nature of his relationships with other people. One of the
best indications of mental health in the adult is a satisfactory marriage—
mind you, I say satisfactory, not happy. Here, as in other departments,
we must not expect too much.

If we have done a reasonably good job of selection, we do not have to
worry about the so-called "accident-prone" person. Any person who is

placed in a system where he doesn't belong might be considered prone to accidents.

If we have been successful in selecting the best man for our system, this is only the beginning. Just as systems, no matter how good they are, break down unattended, so do people. Very good people also get sick, tired, upset, careless, and, inevitably, old. Our biggest errors are not in selection, but in failing to build into our system a periodic review of a man's suitability.

Vested Interest Grows

In the selection process, we give ourselves the right to reject a candidate. But once a man is in the job, as his seniority increases so does his vested interest. As he becomes more convinced about his suitability, we feel less able to challenge it. This is just as true for presidents of corporations as it is for janitors.

The only way to cope with this natural human tendency is to incorporate into the system a way of assessing the changes which overtake people in the psychological as well as in the physical realm. It is no easy thing to evaluate personality change, particularly when we have our own reasons for not wanting to see it. But whether a man has become bitter, resentful, dissatisfied at home and on the job, taken to drink, or succumbed to some slow process of mental deterioration are questions too crucial not to ask.

To summarize what I have tried to say, these are the four factors we need to consider in any program of reducing accidents:

1. A system appropriate to the field of operations
2. Since no system is foolproof, a selection method that will eliminate fools (here defined as people who don't belong in the system), and that will select persons who do fit into the system
3. An ONGOING program of training, drills, checks, count-downs to insure the optimum functioning of the system and the persons in it
4. A method of follow-up and review to improve the system and to consider the suitability of persons in the system

I think all of this is beautifully illustrated in the recent flight of our astronauts. Here we have a machine designed with almost infinite care to meet human requirements, a marvelous system of controls, and a team of men highly selected to meet the most exacting criteria of intelligence, and of physical and psychological health; an extended training period, a system of count-downs to insure that ship and man are in working order, and a method of follow-up.

Man Highly Selected

The men were so highly selected because the system itself could not make all of the decisions. During John Glenn's flight, you will recall that there was a failure in automatic controls regulating the axis of the capsule. There was enough flexibility in controls so that Glenn was able calmly to take over without mishap. As Glenn said about his feelings at this time: "If you're shook up, you shouldn't be there." He should have been there, and he wasn't shook up.

And so, because the system was right, and the man was right, the outcome was predictable—in a word, success. Accident was eliminated because the system had built into it the causes of its own success.

As I consider my remarks, it occurs to me that I have placed great emphasis on how we go about defining words. You might say that I have taken you on an excursion into semantics. This is fine with me so long as you agree that semantics is a matter of utmost importance.

The meaning we give to our words determines the meaning we give to our experience. Our very style of living and behaving is a composite of the meanings we assign to the significant events in our lives. From this point of view, words and their meanings have great power in shaping our destinies.

If we label all of life's unpleasant surprises as accidents, then we come to perceive ourselves as the playthings of fate and we cultivate a philosophy of carelessness and irresponsibility. On the other hand, if we look for causes and hold ourselves accountable for the mishaps in our lives, we become people of resource and confidence, increasingly able to control the direction of events. If these conclusions are as true as I think they are, it matters very much how we define the word accident.

Dangerous Myths

JOYCE DE CICCO

The author dispels some familiar old wives' tales which can lead people who believe in them to injury or death. Although rich in folklore, they sadly lack scientific fact.

How many times have you heard: "A drowning person always comes up three times." "Coffee will sober up a drunk." "A rattlesnake warns before striking." "You should rub snow on frostbite."

Often enough to believe they're true? If so, you're not alone. Nearly everybody, and young people especially, tends to accept these oft-repeated myths as gospel. In reality, however, they're nothing more than old wives' tales, rich in folklore, but sadly lacking in scientific fact.

Acting as though they were literally true is not merely foolish—it can be extremely dangerous. Here are the honest-to-goodness facts about some popular myths that you and your pupils should know to save yourselves from injury or death.

Learn About Lightning

Just because lightning strikes once, don't think you're immune to another flash because of the old adage: Lightning never strikes twice in the same place.

Unfortunately, it does and quite often. Take the case of a young

Reprinted from Joyce de Cicco, "Dangerous Myths," *Safety Education,* XLIII, No. 5 (January 1964), 25–27, by permission of the National Safety Council. Copyright © 1964 by the National Safety Council.

woman in Michigan who dashed from a neighbor's house toward home just as a storm broke. As she reached the middle of the street, the sky crackled and a bolt knocked her down. Her husband, watching through a window, saw her fall and ran to help her. Within seconds, another bolt hit the same spot, striking him too. Both were electrocuted.

"The fact is that if lightning strikes a place once, it is even more likely to seek out the same spot again," says a spokesman for the Lightning Protection Association. "Why? Because lightning prefers the most favorable location, usually the highest point in an area. And a particular place generally remains the highest point for many years."

A classic example is the Empire State Building. It was hit 48 times in one year, and one summer was struck 15 times within 15 minutes!

If it's an average season, about 700 hunters will be killed and 9,000 wounded this year, and a fair percentage will be "safely" attired in the traditional danger color—red. Many hunters put faith in the fallacy that red makes them visible, and is the best color for their clothing.

If you're similarly deluded, consider this teenage hunter in New York. Dressed from head to toe in red, he sat under a tree in open view waiting for the appearance of deer. Another hunter, accompanied by two companions, came up over a slight hill, walked a few paces, then took careful aim and shot the young hunter dead.

Tests made in Massachusetts have proved that red does not show up as well as either yellow or fluorescent orange. Red appears as black at dawn or dusk and can't be distinguished by color-blind hunters. Yellow can be seen a little better, but still doesn't show up as the sun is going down. Best of all is fluorescent orange which stays visible longer after sunset than all other colors and is easier for persons with abnormal vision to see.

With a Silver Spoon . . .

For years, wild mushroom gatherers have been told to give mushrooms the silver spoon or silver coin test. The silver, after coming in contact with a poisonous mushroom, supposedly turns black.

"This test proves nothing except how much sulfur the mushroom contains," says Dr. Everett Beneke, botanist at Michigan State University. He explains that sulfur is what darkens the silver, and that an edible mushroom could contain enough sulfur to turn the spoon, whereas a poisonous mushroom might be low in sulfur and leave the spoon untarnished.

Also, Dr. Beneke advises: Don't place any stock in the superstition that boiling or soaking poisonous mushrooms in salt water makes them safe. That doesn't work either, nor does any simple test. If you don't have the knowledge to distinguish between poisonous and nonpoisonous mushrooms, you shouldn't be picking them.

If you meet a rattlesnake, don't wait for it to shake its tail as a signal of attack before you begin your retreat.

Says zoologist Ray Pawley at Lincoln Park Zoo in Chicago, "A snake doesn't rattle as a sign of aggression, but as a sign of nervousness. Actually, a rattlesnake is afraid of you and uses the sound of its tail to try to frighten you away. If by chance, the tail rattles preceding a strike, it is only a coincidence."

However, if you do hear the dreaded rattle, Pawley says, it is best to walk away quietly and slowly, watching carefully where you step. Don't run; you only excite the snake, making it more apt to strike in self-defense.

Wild Ideas About Water

It's amazing how many people have dangerous ideas about water and drowning. In a recent survey of sixth-graders, 44 percent of them thought you should jump in the water to save a drowning person; 38 percent said it is impossible to stay afloat in water for long with clothes on, and that if a boat overturns you should swim to shore, and 31 percent believed a drowning person comes up three times.

"The worst thing you can do is dive in after a floundering swimmer," says the American Red Cross. "Too often, the would-be rescuer drowns while the victim in trouble swims safely to shore—or the drowning person struggles and gets a vise-like grip on the rescuer's neck and they both go down."

Don't Drown Yourself

Proper procedure for rescuing a drowning person, according to the Red Cross is: Throw the victim something buoyant to stay afloat on—a buoy, life jacket, beach ball, hunk of wood. Or extend to him a pole, your shirt and, as a last resort, your hands.

As for staying up with clothes on, it's entirely possible if you don't panic. Shipwrecked sailors during World War II were known to bob along on ocean waves, fully clothed, for as long as eight hours. Sometimes you can blow air into your clothes, making them serve as makeshift life preservers.

And try to make it to shore after a boat capsizes? *Never,* say experts. Even good swimmers underestimate the distance, become exhausted and sink. Best policy is "stick with the ship." It will float, keeping you safe until rescue.

As for that old superstition that a drowning person surfaces three times before he goes down for the last and fatal time—there's absolutely nothing to it, say lifesaving authorities. Many drowning victims sink like rocks and never reappear. Some struggle and thrash to the surface a dozen times.

Facts About Floundering Swimmers

Why and how often a drowning person comes up is explained in the Red Cross Lifesaving Manual:

> If a person loses his tidal air (normal amount breathed) on the first downward trip and can make no move to rise again he will not of his own volition reappear at the surface. On the other hand, if he managed to hold some tidal air on each downward trip and can make frantic clawing efforts to return to the surface, the chances are he will reappear not once or thrice, but perhaps half a dozen times.

Unless you're up to date in first-aid methods, you may still falsely assume that a tourniquet is the best way to stop bleeding. It definitely is not. The tourniquet stops the flow of blood through a limb, and if left on for a mere 15 minutes can sometimes damage the tissue, resulting in gangrene and loss of the limb.

Authorities now unanimously reject the tourniquet's use except in very severe cases, such as when a limb is crushed or severed. Otherwise, the recommended way to stop bleeding is to put direct pressure on the wound after covering it with a clean cloth.

On the subject of first-aid fallacies: Were you ever advised to put butter on a burn, beef steak on a black eye or wound, a cold knife on a bump on the head or to blow smoke in the ear of a person with an earache? All of these are popular home remedies without any healing effect, says Dr. Marie A. Hinrichs, of the American Medical Association.

"They probably originated because, being soothing or cold, they relieve some discomfort and make the victim feel better," she says. "But they don't really do any good and are unsanitary."

Another fantastic first-aid misconception that authorities abhor is that you should rub snow on frostbite. "Where this absurdity ever got started, I can't imagine," says Clint Hoch, first-aid expert for the National Safety Council. "Making frozen tissue even colder by applying snow is against all common sense. And rubbing cold, numbed skin could cause an abrasion and the victim wouldn't realize it. In extreme cases, gangrene could result."

How to Treat Frostbite

Thawing out the frozen tissue by warming it up gradually is the only sane procedure, recommends Hoch. Get the victim into a warm room, apply blankets and have him drink warm liquids. But don't apply direct heat; it may burn the insensitive tissue.

Dramatists have been mainly responsible for spreading the false idea that the primary danger from leaking gas is asphyxiation. How many television and movie suicides have you seen accomplished by turning on the gas in the oven? It's often phony. Breathing enough of the gas to cause death is possible, but is very difficult, says Hans Grigo of NSC's Home Department. The gas is not poisonous, he explains. To kill, it must dilute the normal 20 percent concentration of oxygen in the air, reducing the amount available to you. And this can take a long time. Many people overlook the big danger of escaping gas—explosion. Dozens of homes are destroyed this way every year.

Why Coffee Won't Sober Him

A fable believed by nearly everyone is that coffee will help sober up a drunk. But it's just not true.

According to recent studies on alcohol and coffee done by Dr. R. B. Forney at Indiana University Medical School, coffee has no sobering effect. There is no ingredient in coffee that will alleviate the effects of alcohol. "The only advantage to drinking coffee," says Dr. Forney, "is to prevent the intake of more alcohol and delay a person from driving until some of the alcohol is eliminated from his system. But a cold glass of water would do the same thing."

Do you believe smaller vehicles can stop in less time and distance than larger ones? Seems logical maybe, but tests show it's not so, according to Robert L. Donigan of Northwestern University's Traffic Institute.

But there is some truth in this misconception when it comes to heavily loaded semi-trailer trucks, admits Donigan. They don't stop as soon, but not because of their size or weight. It's because the brakes won't lock the wheels when the vehicle is heavily loaded, or the driver is afraid to lock them for fear of jackknifing.

And do you think that pumping your brakes helps you stop more quickly? Most people do. But here again they're wrong, says the Traffic Institute. "Experiments show that a driver can stop in considerably less distance on dry pavement by holding his brake pedal down than by pumping." However, National Safety Council experts recommend pumping your brakes to stop on snow or ice-covered pavement. By pumping your brakes, the front wheels roll between applications, letting you retain steering control of your car.

Clearing your pupils' minds of these dangerous misconceptions is important. For, as safety experts have proved, what you don't know *can* hurt you.

Oh, Who Cares About Safety?

JAMES R. ADAMS

Some thought-provoking comments are given concerning why it is that people don't care much about safety or about being careful. No single panacea is offered although the author feels that progress will come slowly in diminishing the magnitude of the accident problem.

Nobody *wants* to be hurt. Obviously then, people should *want* to be *safe*. But it isn't quite that easy. As you well know, motivating people for accident prevention is a hard job. It is safety's major problem. Why?

I wish I had a simple answer. I wish I could say: "Here is the pill for what ails you. Take it and you will get well." But I can't. In safety, the simple answers were discovered long ago. Any improvements at this stage of the game will be hard to come by, and if you long for easy panaceas for this problem of motivating people, you will find little assurance in the points of view I have to offer.

What Is an Accident?

Let's start by defining our terms. We aim at reducing the number and severity of accidents. Well then, what is an accident?

By an accident we generally mean an event which is *unintended, unexpected,* and which *hurts* somebody. Accidents are caused—and the cause, more often than not, involves an action by the victim himself. But

Reprinted from James R. Adams, "Oh, Who Cares About Safety?" *Safety Education,* XLII, No. 5 (January 1963), 7–8, by permission of the National Safety Council. Copyright © 1963 by the National Safety Council.

while accidents have causes, it is seldom that these causes are readily apparent to the victim or to anyone else prior to the accident. We are seldom able to foresee with *certainty* that an injurious event will occur; we see rather that there is a *probability* that it might occur.

This uncertainty is fundamental to the accident problem. Accidents occur very infrequently to any one person, and the probability of an accident at any given time is *very low*. In fact, the probability is so slight that for many people it loses any sense of reality—certainly any sense of urgency. So there develops a feeling that accidents happen only to other people. And of course, the fact of the matter is that accidents do happen to other people—almost always.

The Odds Are Against Us

Now, this matter of *probability* is closely linked up with the question of *cost*. Let me illustrate: When you flip a coin to see who will pay for coffee, your probability of winning isn't very good—you are as likely to lose as to win. But if you lose, the cost of losing is very slight. So you don't worry about flipping for coffee, even though the odds aren't favorable.

But take a look at another situation, one in which the elements are reversed. In a little stunt known as "Russian Roulette," the odds of losing are much reduced—one in five. But while the odds of losing are much less, the *cost* of losing is infinitely greater. It is, quite literally, "infinite"— you lose your life.

In facing the problem of accidents, we are up against a situation comparable in this regard to Russian Roulette. The probability of an accident is very low—but the cost of an accident may be very great. It may also be infinite.

In order to deal with such a situation, a person needs to be strongly motivated. To sustain a constant safety consciousness day in and day out, year in and year out, against the very unlikely possibility of an accident, calls for strong and abiding motivation. And it is here, I believe, that we fall short.

Your own experience will testify—and accident statistics will confirm— that in many people, there is insufficient motivation to live safely. Why is this so?

What About Self-preservation?

First of all, the very existence of a problem in safety motivation is, in itself, a convincing argument against the notion that people are motivated by an "instinct of self preservation." We have no such instinct. We are not born with any built-in mechanism which keeps us safety-conscious in the conditions of modern civilized existence. What we *are* born with is an ability to learn. And we either learn to want to be safe, or we fail to learn to want to be safe.

We have already noted that the low frequency of accidents allows a sense of personal security—a feeling that "It won't happen to me."

In addition, there is the all-too-human tendency to avoid thinking about whatever is *unpleasant*. It is this tendency that leads to what Freud has called the "invulnerability of the hero"—the hero, of course, being oneself. Each man is the hero of his own daydreams, and in our daydreams we always escape *unhurt* from every predicament. In our daydreams we never die. To be hurt or to die is an unpleasant thought; and we tend to avoid dwelling on that which is unpleasant.

The mere thought of having an accident also is unpleasant. And, finding the thought distasteful, we tend to push it from our minds and so do not attend it. Our unwillingness to face up to the unpleasantness of the prospect of accidents is part of the reason that we lack sufficient motivation to prevent them.

Part of Another Problem

Another aspect of the problem of safety motivation comes into play when the accident hazard is bound up with some *other* problem for which we have found no solution. Take, for example, the accidents known as slips and falls.

In many of the injury reports, there appear such phrases as: "His leg gave way," or "Her foot failed to support her." Sometimes this represents a physical infirmity, but in many such cases, I am convinced that the accidents follow from lack of proper exercise. Falls are a symptom of the much larger problem of how to get the exercise that nature requires of us—in spite of the fact that working and learning are usually sedentary occupations.

It should be apparent that solving a problem will be more difficult if that problem exists as a solution to some other problem. For example, suppose that Mr. X wants to quit smoking because he is afraid of lung cancer. But when he cuts down his smoking, his weight increases. It will be harder for him to give up smoking because it serves as part of the solution to the problem of controlling his weight.

In the matter of slips and falls, I think we have a similar situation. When a woman goes out into the "man's world" of business, she wants to make certain that her femininity is not reduced as a consequence. So she insists on wearing high-heeled shoes which give inadequate support for walking, and contribute in large measure to the fact that women fall so often.

Adolescent boys, insecure about their status as adults, often "prove" their masculinity by taking daring, dangerous chances. They think of safety precautions as "sissified" and unmanly. Here again, the unsafe behavior which causes accident problems exists as a solution to some other problem. You must solve one to fight the other.

The "Chip-away" Philosophy

In summary, inadequate motivation to safety seems to be related to the low frequency of accidents to the individual, to the unpleasantness of the thought of getting hurt, and to the fact that accident hazards often exist in association with some other problem for which no solution has been found that is both safe and acceptable.

These difficulties are present all the time. There is no escaping them any more than there is any escape from the possibility of accident.

I don't want to end on a note of pessimism or hopelessness. I do not personally feel that the prospects are hopeless. On the other hand, I do not see any grand and simple answer—any dramatic breakthroughs. I do not anticipate a Salk vaccine for unsafe people.

But there is much that can be accomplished by steadily working away at the problem. I am firmly committed to the "chip-away" philosophy of safety. Progress will come as we chip away at the difficulties bit by bit, and thus slowly diminish the magnitude of the problem.

I am further convinced that the effort is very worthwhile. The probability of accidents may be low, but the cost is much, much too high.

Strategies for Cutting Highway Losses

WILLIAM HADDON, JR.

ALBERT BENJAMIN KELLEY

Although this article discusses strategies for dealing with highway losses, implications of the three strategies presented may be applied to many accident types. Examples of countermeasures involve many safety activities. The authors suggest a priority; one of the three strategies should be emphasized for reducing highway accident losses.

Three basic strategies shape successful programs to counteract the human and economic loss that occurs when people and their property come into physical conflict with natural or manmade hazards in the environment.

In countless day-to-day sorts of activity, these three strategies are employed in one mix or another—by doctors, public health officers, engineers, and insurers—to hold down and in some cases completely eliminate losses occurring when man's interests collide with his environment. Their applications have extended across programs to protect people and property from the hazards of storms, floods, harnessed power such as electricity and nuclear energy, infection, transportation and contaminated water and air.

Preventing Contact

The first strategy is to lower the frequency with which people or their property connect with manmade hazards. Many tactics long in use attempt this.

Among these, some seek to eliminate the hazard by, for example, legislating against fireworks, guns and nuclear bombs, or for pasteurization of milk and chlorination of water to eliminate hazardous organisms.

Some modify the hazard, such as by seeding hurricanes, slowing aircraft landing and ground vehicle speeds, blowing off steam with safety valves, using safer voltages, using tempered glass in doors and panels, reducing the maximum temperature of household hot water, rounding the edges and corners of toys and buildings, and diluting or altering hazardous chemicals for shipment.

Some separate, in either space or time, the susceptible people and structures from the hazard, through use of pedestrian overpasses, traffic lights, electrical and thermal insulation, buried or elevated electrical cables, non- or restricted-licensing of dangerous drivers, alerts and evacuations anticipating earthquakes, storms, and floods, other warnings—"dangerous curves," "hazardous voltage," "polluted water—no swimming," "moving machinery"—and separation of sources of heat from explosives and flammables.

Still others seek hazard recognition and avoidance through formal coursework such as driver education. First strategy approaches in the case of highway loss reduction appear to offer limited additional payoffs in the years immediately ahead.

Softening Contact

The second strategy is to soften the interaction of the environmental hazard and people or structures once they come in contact, whether or not because of human error.

Here, too, many tactics have long been in use. The seismographs that automatically stop the Japanese high-speed trains when tremors reach given force levels are an interesting example. Others include flood dikes, sunburn preventives, fuses, rollbars, hard hats, boxing gloves, safety shoes, lead x-ray shields, blast and fallout shelters, fire sprinkler systems and doors, nets for acrobats, and fire nets.

It has been known since the early 1940s that many driver and passenger deaths and severe injuries could be eliminated under this strategy by the use of damage-reducing principles similar to those long employed in freight packaging. Yet until recently, traditional emphasis in highway safety has been placed almost exclusively on crash prevention. Currently, however, the utility of this strategy to highway loss reduction objectives is being illustrated by, for instance, crash helmets, safety belts, breakaway sign posts, laminated windshields that act like fire nets on impact, structures placed in some cars to resist lateral impact, and energy-absorbing steering columns.

Air bag technology and impact-absorbing bumper innovations have high potential for softening the damaging interaction of people and property with the forces at play on our highways. And developments in such areas as damage-resistant materials and structures for car exteriors hold promise for sizable injury and property damage amelioration if they are vigorously encouraged by industry elements with a stake in the outcome. Writers of codes for structural resistance to fire, wind, and earthquakes have always known that property with a high likelihood of exposure to impact forces—such as automobiles—can be designed and built to withstand many expected environmental assaults with little or no economic penalty.

Post-Contact Aid

The third strategy is to detect, signal, and salvage threatened people and property in the face of damage already done.

Some practices under this strategy are concerned with early detection. Transducers on aircraft and helicopters that start broadcasting a special signal at time of a crash are an example, as are fire and theft signaling systems, MAYDAY and SOS signals and the use of forest fire towers. Other tactics involve evaluating the alerting message, dispatching a competent and timely response—such as an ambulance helicopter in a war zone— and retrieval of damaged people and property as typified by Coast Guard rescue operations. Still others provide alongside emergency fire and medical services at airport runways.

The potential offered by this strategy for highway loss reduction remains largely untapped. Huge improvements are possible in emergency medical care services, including onsite, in-transit and in-hospital emergency treatment, and in the communications systems which trigger emergency medical care into action in response to a crash. In the area of property loss, salvaging techniques to speed removal of crash debris— thereby reducing the possibility of new crashes being caused by the wreckage of old ones—must be developed. So must a dependable system to identify roadside obstacles that have contributed to crash severity so that they can be removed or modified.

Can Accidents Be Managed?

WALTER H. KOHL

The author raises this all-important question and describes several categories of accidents. He states that the attitude of people towards accidents is the single crucial factor in accident control.

In 1967, the death toll in U.S.A. from all types of accidents was 112,000. The accumulated loss to the economy amounted to $21.3 billion, according to figures released by the National Safety Council. Accidents on the highways killed 53,100 people in 1967, and the cost of this toll is estimated at nearly $11 billion. One observer states that if fatalities from motor-car accidents continue to increase at the rate established between 1961 and 1964, they will reach the awesome figure of 200,000 by 1984.

It has been said frequently that we live in an economy of waste, and consume our resources at a faster rate than we can afford. The material loss resulting from accidents in general may be a small fraction of the total waste, and therefore easily sustained. But should we stand idly by while the loss of lives continues to increase? It can hardly be our intent to counteract the population explosion in this manner. To close our eyes to the untold suffering of the bereaved and of those who have been crippled for life would in Christian society be an indefensible attitude.

A number of private and public agencies are concerned with this problem, but their efforts have not been able to stem the tide. The National Safety Council is able to predict that a certain number of deaths

Reprinted from Walter H. Kohl, "Can Accidents Be Managed?" *Journal of the American Society of Safety Engineers*, XIII, No. 11 (November 1968), 10–12, by permission of the American Society of Safety Engineers. Copyright © 1968 by the American Society of Safety Engineers. Footnotes have been renumbered.

will occur, but its warnings seem to have no effect. The casualty figures continue to rise from year to year. People refuse to be scared by statistics. There ought to be some way by which the toll from accidents in general can be managed more effectively.

Since this country prides itself in its management ability, it would seem proper to launch a large-scale effort to manage accidents. A public venture, such as "Accident Prevention, Incorporated," should be succesful, as every citizen is a risk and therefore no doubt anxious to become a shareholder. Such an organization would differ from an insurance company by paying hidden dividends in terms of safety, rather than paying damages for sustained accidents.

Before pursuing this concept, it would be well to state what are usually considered to be the main features of management, determine the make-up of accidents, and then investigate whether their control can properly be approached from a management point of view.

Management is concerned with the coordination of multiple efforts. It is true that an individual may manage his own affairs, but Management with a capital 'M' relates to many people who are directed to perform certain tasks, so that a large-scale objective can be reached. In business, a corporate enterprise aims at a profit for its shareholders and achieves this end by rendering a useful service, or by manufacturing a product for which the public is willing to pay a reasonable price.

A government agency or research institution, while not concerned with the profit motive, nevertheless must operate within an assigned budget, and needs good management to perform effectively in its prescribed function. The people involved in any such enterprise must be motivated properly and rewarded adequately for their efforts. All kinds of material, equipment, and machinery may be needed in the operation. To function smoothly, both the people and the equipment must be controlled, and safeguards provided against undisciplined behavior or breakdown.

Our industrial civilization operates essentially within this framework, and the high standards of living enjoyed by so many of its participants bears witness to its effectiveness. However, the various social ailments from which we still suffer are an indication that we have not "managed" our affairs to the best of our ability in all areas. Accidents are unquestionably one of these ailments.

The Make-Up of Accidents

Several categories of accidents exist, and they may be described under the following headings:

Accidents caused by the victim's own negligence
—by the victim's lack of alertness
—by the negligence of others and their lack of alertness
—by faulty equipment
—by catastrophic events.

In all five categories, we are confronted with an unexpected event that causes us harm or loss of property. It should be noted that the results of crime and vandalism are the same as those of accidents. However, the purposeful, damaging acts of misguided people are not of concern in this discussion.

1. Accidents caused by the victim's own negligence are very common; many of these can be avoided by using ordinary caution, or by observing prescribed safety regulations. Driving in a heavy snowstorm, or in a thick fog, is asking for trouble. Operating machine tools without using the prescribed protective gear is foolish and has nothing to do with superior skill or long-term experience. Many more such examples could be cited. Some people, especially the young, like to live dangerously and refuse to appraise the risks. Immaturity is probably a common characteristic of all offenders in this category, young and old alike.

2. Accidents caused by the victim's lack of alertness are set apart from those caused by negligence, because no conscious offense of existing safety regulations is involved in this case. It is more a matter of being absent-minded. Some months ago, I pulled down a garage door with my fingers by putting them into the gaps between the horizontal boards, neglecting to use the handle provided for this purpose. The boards closed down on my finger tips like the jaws of a vise, until I pulled the door up again with my free hand. The results were painful, to say the least. On the other hand, I have never seen a sign forbidding such stupid action, and it might not have done any good if one had been posted. If one's mind is not on the task at hand, signs are ignored. The designer of the door should have thought of this possible abuse. Overlapping guard strips would make such folding doors safe, especially for children and absent-minded professors.

To prevent accidents of this kind requires considerable mental discipline, i.e., continuous presence of mind and quick response to unforeseen situations. The cultivation of such safety consciousness should be part of the educational process in schools.

3. Accidents caused by the negligence of others and by their lack of alertness: Many accidents on the highways lead to injury or death of people who did not themselves offend any safety rules but who became victims of the irresponsible action of others. The continuous exposure

of a cautious driver to this type of hazard is one of the most frightening aspects of highway travel. It is good advice always to be prepared for the car ahead doing exactly the opposite to what its turning light indicates, and to assume that the driver of another car did not see your own signal.

4. Accidents caused by faulty equipment: It should not be too difficult to make substantial progress in the elimination of unsafe equipment and of defective materials. Ensuring public safety is a government function that is performed most effectively when it has the whole-hearted support of the public, of manufacturers, trade organizations, and professional societies, all of whom should contribute to the enactment and enforcement of safety regulations that aim at the production of reliable equipment.

Equipment and materials which are initially sound will deteriorate in in time by wear and corrosion, and will become unsafe. Regular inspection can uncover such incipient faults, as shown in industry, in public housing, in mines, and indeed in motor vehicles.

When an article or device has become the personal property of an individual and is used only by him, or within his family, inspection and repair is left to the user's discretion; it cannot be enforced. The children's toys may threaten to fall apart, rusty nails be in evidence, and electric wiring become defective; all of which may cause serious accidents unless remedied quickly.

5. Accidents caused by catastrophic events, such as fire, lightning, or earthquakes, can be minimized only if one has learned to take the proper steps long before such events occur. To keep doors and windows closed in case of fire is not a natural reaction, but requires some mental preparation. In many such cases, there is no defense at all. If a plane crashes in a residential area, disaster strikes without warning. On the other hand, when the driver of a school bus (Boyd Jones [1] of Harvard, Ill.) became aware of an approaching tornado, stopped the vehicle, and ordered his 20 charges to lie in a ditch beside the road, he demonstrated what can be done to outwit natural disaster.

The Management of Accidents

It must now be asked which of the causes of accident are subject to control and what forms such controls must take to be effective. Negligence, lack of alertness, faulty equipment, and catastrophic events were the main causes of accidents in the different categories that were discussed here. Of these, faulty or unsafe equipment presents an essentially technical prob-

[1] *Boston Globe:* (April 22, 1967).

lem, although it was noted that the human element entered into this category when it came to the proper maintenance of equipment. Negligence and lack of alertness seem to be decisive factors in all categories.

It appears, then, that we cannot fully control and therefore manage accidents without extending our sphere of influence to embrace the attitude of people, especially of those who either lack a sense of social responsibility or who find it difficult to foresee the results of their actions. Such an extension of control is bound to have vast socioeconomic implications, as will here become apparent.

A study conducted by Goen [2] at Stanford Research Institute shows that traffic fatalities, to consider just one area, could be reduced by 90 percent, saving 45,000 lives on the basis of the 1965 fatality rate, if the following measures were taken:

1. Refuse driving privileges to those under 21 or over 70 years of age, as well as to five percent of the remainder who have twice the average accident rate.
2. Reduce speed limits by 20 percent and introduce automated systems for the enforcement of penalties for violations.
3. Provide for one-way traffic and grade-separated intersections on highways, as well as for overpasses for pedestrians on urban arterials by allocating $10 billion per year for safety improvements in the road system.
4. Enforce safe design of automobiles.
5. Develop high-speed intercity ground transport and rapid-transit systems so as to largely eliminate the use of automobiles for commuting and intercity travel.

The SRI Report faces the facts as they exist and addresses itself to the problem of reducing the slaughter on the highways by suggesting commendable measures on the technical plane (items 2 to 5) and highly restrictive legislation for young and old people alike. Item 1, above, would remove 20 million drivers from the roads. Needless to say, the effects of such action on the motorcar industry and on the insurance business would be severe.

It is very unlikely that lawmakers would take on the burden of enacting legislation that would put such drastic measures into effect. The halls of the legislature would resound with the screams of millions of people who are affected adversely by these regulations. But then, not all elderly people are safety risks and not all teenagers are irresponsible. Some distinc-

2 R. L. Goen: Drastic Measures for Reducing Traffic Casualties, Stanford Research Institute, Menlo Park, Calif. (Dec. 1965).

tion should be made on the basis of health records and performance. Attempts to formalize such controls of driving privileges indiscriminately at suggested age levels would be a serious mistake.

On the other hand, it must be realized that attempts to modify the attitude of drivers by persuasion and education have not been successful. On this basis, one wonders whether self-protection will not in the end force the public to accept even such drastic measures as pulling 20 million drivers off the road.

The basic issue, on which our entire argument in this article hinges, is to make safety acceptable to human beings so that they will consciously strive for it and accept certain sacrifices to achieve it. We face the same problem when discussing war and peace, which are extensions of accidents and safety onto a global scale. Ferre [3] has pointed out in a searching analysis that men do not want peace because war offers an escape from the meaninglessness and boredom of life, a relief from fear and frustration. He calls for "effective motivation for universal meanings, a new sense of self and of self-regard both for the person and for the nation" as a prescription for peace. Following this line of reasoning, it will be necessary to make safety meaningful. To motivate people so that they will take safety to heart will require a deeper appreciation of the common weal in which the value of the individual life merges with that of the "commonwealth."

Negligence would then become an offense that would weigh more heavily on the individual's conscience; it would become a religious issue. In a similar vein, Wharton [4] emphasized the need for applying the now-available methods of psychiatry to the correction of man's propensity to enact and condone mass killing. And Tinbergen [5] points out that "a scientific understanding of our behavior, leading to its control, may well be the most urgent task that faces mankind today."

It may be said in conclusion that the management of accidents, as somewhat glibly proposed at the beginning of this discussion, is a myth, because this concept does not strike at the core of the problem. Building more reliable devices, safer cars, better highways, is all to the good, but as one observer said, "it is similar to the attempt of reducing the occurrence of crime by making it harder to steal, or to kill, rather than by improving the social climate." The attitude of people is the basic issue. This attitude cannot be managed, but only improved slowly by the individual's acceptance of a different set of values. As man is the only species that is a mass murderer, "the only misfit in his own society," [6] we may have to turn to the animals to find a way out of our dilemma.

[3] N. S. Ferre: Does Man Really Want Peace? *Saturday Review,* (July 1, 1967).
[4] John F. Wharton: En Route to a Massacre? *Saturday Review,* (Nov. 4, 1967).
[5] N. Tinbergen: On War and Peace in Animals and Man, *Science,* Vol. 160 (June 28, 1968), pp. 1411–1418.
[6] *Ibid.*

The Influence of Societal Values on Rates of Death and Injury

DAVID KLEIN

The thesis of this article states that a significant proportion of accidents are the inevitable result of a discrepancy between cultural demands and social and technological reality. The author makes a pessimistic prediction that, as a result of this discrepancy, accident losses in number and rates will continue to rise regardless of countermeasures developed. However, he also suggests action to take for preventing accidental injury and death.

If an incurable optimist were to search for trends of the 1960's that might help him predict accident morbidity and mortality in the 1970's, he would probably find some grounds for optimism. He might note, for example, the following developments, all of which occurred during the decade of the 1960's:

1. A substantial increase in both money and manpower devoted to research in injury control—and greater sophistication in their deployment;
2. An upsurge of concern with ecology—a concern that inevitably encompasses a wide variety of environmental hazards;
3. A general increase in what has come to be called "consumerism" —a movement that seems likely to concern itself with the inherent hazards built into products as well as with shoddiness in their manufacture and fraud in their distribution;
4. The assumption of an active role by the federal government with

Reprinted from David Klein, "The Influence of Societal Values on Rates of Death and Injury," *Journal of Safety Research*, III, No. 1 (March 1971), 2–8, by permission of the National Safety Council. Copyright © 1971 by the National Safety Council.

respect to product safety—in the establishment not only of a Commission on Product Safety but, probably more important, the National Highway Safety Bureau, with power to specify safety features of new automobiles and to institute recall of models that prove unsafe;

5. An attempt at gun-control legislation, which, though minimal, provides a basis for further legislation.

But optimists tend to read data superficially and selectively. A more objective attempt at prediction would take note of the following trends, which were equally apparent during the past decade:

1. Highway deaths increased—and the horse-power rating of the average passenger car almost doubled;
2. Firearms deaths increased sharply—as did the private ownership of firearms, especially hand guns;
3. Private aircraft fatalities increased sharply;
4. Several new recreational devices—notably, trampolines, snowmobiles, and mini-bikes—were widely accepted by the public and made large and increasing contributions to mortality and morbidity;
5. The proliferation of home power tools—power mowers, home workshops, chain saws—also added to the injury data.

In brief, if these trends continue through the next decade, the prediction must be rather pessimistic: accidental injury and death are likely to increase significantly, both in absolute numbers and in rates, despite the countermeasures that have been developed.

The reasons for this prediction are several. To begin with, most of the control measures that our optimist has singled out are "post mortem" in nature. That is, they require that a certain amount of morbidity and mortality actually occur before a specific product or environmental hazard comes to notice. And substantially more morbidity and mortality will inevitably occur before a countermeasure or a regulatory mechanism can be established and made operational. The snowmobile offers an interesting example. Hundreds of deaths occurred in the past two years before the lethality of this device came to public attention and hundreds more will occur next winter while regulatory agencies are pondering effective countermeasures.

One study of injury control (Bhise and Rockwell, 1968) has compared this process to that of a man taking a shower under a shower head located fifty feet from the shower controls. By the time he has completed the 100-foot round trip to adjust the controls, the situation at the shower head may well have changed. But this analogy disregards the fact that in injury control the fifty-foot path is blocked by two high, and often impassable, hurdles.

One of the hurdles consists, of course, of the special-interest groups that oppose and resist safety regulations—the automobile manufacturers who for years have testified in Washington that certain safety features are technically unfeasible or inordinately expensive; the gun users and the gun pushers, who have very effectively defeated legislation for realistic gun control; the private pilots who lobby against restrictions on personal aircraft; the motorcyclists and manufacturers who for a time successfully opposed the compulsory helmet law.

But, as we have seen frequently in the past, special-interest groups can be defeated by the force of outraged public opinion. Why then, does injury control, in terms of both research and regulation, remain at the level of tokenism? The answer to this question brings us to the second high hurdle: American cultural values. There are several reasons why Americans *do not want* as safe an environment as could be achieved with our existing technical knowledge and our current level of political process. And the reasons behind this tolerance of—if not actual desire for—risk and danger represent another trend (ignored by our optimist) that became more pronounced during the 1960's. This is the growing discrepancy between the cultural values and the social reality. This discrepancy seems likely to generate far more injuries than the trends toward injury control can prevent.

Cultural Demands vs. Social and Technological Realities

Whenever a society's values and beliefs lag seriously behind its current social and technological realities, social pathology is likely to occur. Many of India's current problems, for example, can be traced to beliefs and values about land-holding, child-bearing, and the environment in general that are not functional in a society faced with a rising population and an insufficient food supply. In the United States today, there is a similar lag between values and reality—and this lag leads to, among other things, accidental injury and death.

Despite our society's obvious and irreversible trends toward urbanization, greater industrialization, and greater population density, and despite the increasing societal interdependence that these changes demand, many of the values taught by the schools and reinforced by the mass media still reflect the needs of a frontier society. Our children, like ourselves, are taught very early and very effectively:

1. That competitiveness of a rather aggressive type is individually useful and socially desirable;
2. That individual initiative and independence of action lead to success;
3. That one should seek maximal individual autonomy and control over one's environment;
4. That masculinity implies toughness, aggressiveness, and the ability to withstand stress;
5. That challenge and excitement should be actively sought, and that risk-taking is justified in the meeting of challenge;
6. That status and other social rewards are more readily earned through individual achievement than through cooperative, group effort.

These are the values taught by teachers and textbooks. They are the values exemplified by our cultural heroes, historical, fictional, and contemporary. They are the values reinforced continuously by the mass media. And thus they become cultural demands—with which everyone must comply if he is to gain self-respect, acceptance, and status in our society.

In a frontier society, individual initiative, aggressive competition, risk-taking, and the ability to withstand stress, *when exercised in the sphere of production,* promote not only the survival of the individual but the economic welfare of the society as a whole. The United States could not have achieved, in a mere two centuries, its economic and technological leadership had not numberless individuals been willing to meet challenge, behave aggressively, and take risk—in exploring new territory, exploiting natural resources, inventing new machines, founding new enterprises.

But a highly industrialized society, by its very nature, minimizes risk-taking and stress, and routinizes work by dividing it into smaller and smaller repetitive segments. Thus it concentrates major decision-making—and hence control over the environment—into fewer and fewer hands. Fewer and fewer workers, whether they wear blue collars or white, can exercise (or can feel that they exercise) in their work such cultural values as initiative, individual ingenuity, risk-taking, or aggressiveness. Fewer and fewer of them can gain from their work a sense of power, individual achievement, or control over the environment.

Some behavioral scientists (e.g., Thompson and Van Houten, 1970) classify occupations as either *discretionary* or *routine*. The discretionary occupation requires that the worker make a variety of individual decisions which culminate in the task's being done well or badly; thus it offers him some opportunity to gain distinction through using the cultural values, since individual initiative or sound risk-taking or sheer competitiveness can result in his doing the job in a new and superior way.

The routine occupation, on the other hand, has each of its component tasks so carefully specified and prescribed that the worker cannot possibly achieve distinction or status. He either does the job correctly—as it is prescribed—or he fails at it. There is almost no way, for example, in which an assembly-line worker or a lab technician or a bank clerk or an air traffic controller or a junior computer programmer or a middle-level executive can achieve distinction or a sense of personal power in his work situation through risk-taking, competitiveness, individual initiative, etc.

But since he has been taught that he *should* compete, take risks, master his environment, show initiative, etc., and since he cannot fulfill these cultural demands in his work situation, he is virtually forced to fulfill them in the sphere of consumption rather than production—that is, in activities centered in the home and in recreational activities. Thus, although he cannot achieve status by developing a new work process or by demonstrating individual skill and daring on the job, he can achieve it by designing a bookshelf in his basement workshop, by shooting a twelve-point deer, by winning a snowmobile or motorcycle race, by becoming a sky-diver, or by flying a private airplane.

Whether or not the proportion of routine to discretionary occupations is increasing is difficult to determine. The recent increases in economic concentration in the form of corporate mergers and the proliferation of automation would seem to have reduced the number of discretionary occupations—though reliable data are difficult to come by. But whether or not routine occupations are on the increase, two further developments are unquestionable: First, increasing affluence enables the routine worker to surround himself with a wide array of increasingly powerful recreational devices—power tools, outboard boats, high performance cars, snowmobiles, etc.—all of which, in fact or in fantasy, offer him the feelings of control, power, "masculinity," and risk which no longer are available at work. Secondly, the steady reduction in the length of the work week gives the routine worker time in which to use these devices and, hence, a justification for buying them. And this, in turn, motivates the manufacturer to produce an ever-increasing variety of such devices and, by stressing the "excitement" and "thrill" they offer (e.g., in the advertisements for snowmobiles), to persuade the potential customer that he genuinely wants them.

All of this is relevant to accidental injury for two reasons. First, since almost all injury is caused by the uncontrolled transfer of energy to the body (Haddon, 1970; Haddon, Suchman, and Klein, 1964), the more sources of potential energy in the environment, the greater the likelihood of injury. But even more important is the fact that the devices we have mentioned are used not in an industrial environment, which can be—and to a large extent has been—accident-proofed, but in a domestic or recreational environment which is infinitely more difficult to accident-proof. It is far easier, for example, to install fail-safe switches on a potentially dangerous machine or to persuade a lathe operator to wear safety goggles than to prevent a hunter or motorcyclist from using unsafe equipment or from behaving unsafely.

This is not sheer speculation. As Figure 8–1 demonstrates, the rate of increase in several categories of nonindustrial fatalities has, during the 1960's, far exceeded the rate of increase of the population. It can be argued, of course, that the data in Figure 8–1 have not been "corrected for exposure"—that the fatality rate per 100,000 firearms or per 1,000,000 passenger miles flown in private aircraft has not increased so sharply or may in fact have decreased. But this argument ignores the fundamentally relevant question: What are the cultural forces that cause people to acquire guns and snowmobiles and to expose themselves to risk in the air and on the highway?

Figure 8–2 illustrates only one example of the increase in mechanical power available to the individual during this period. And the same

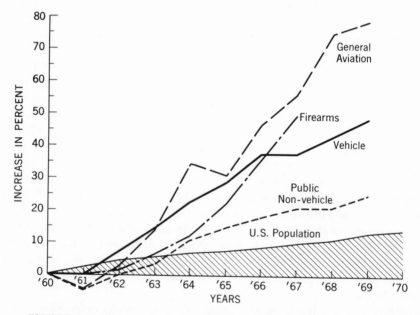

FIGURE 8–1   *Increase in Fatal Injuries vs. Increase in Population 1960–1969.* *(Comparable data for firearms fatalities after 1967 are not yet available. The data presented include homicidal deaths since these, like "gunshot accidents," are always unintended from the point of view of the victim and often unintended from the point of view of the perpetrator, and since they would not have occurred had not a high-energy source in the form of a firearm been available.)* **Sources: Accident Facts, Vital Statistics of the United States, and Statistical Abstract of the United States.**

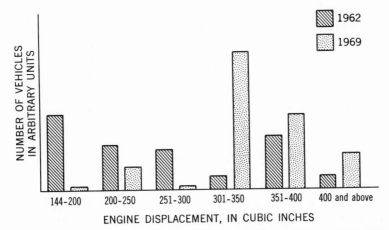

FIGURE 8-2   Horsepower of U.S. Passenger Vehicles 1962 vs. 1969. This increase in horsepower is not, of course, directly related to the increase in the fatality rate, since part of the horsepower increment is used to move heavier vehicles or to operate such accessories as air conditioners. Nevertheless, the loss experience reported by casualty insurance companies in connection with so-called "high-performance" cars lends support to the possibility that such a relationship does, in fact, exist. Source: **Ward's Automotive Yearbook.**

decade saw a steady trend in the development of new devices that offered nothing functional other than a sense of excitement or risk—the racing go-kart, the trampoline, the trail bike, the snowmobile, the sky-diver's parachute, the water skier's kite. By the time the morbidity resulting from any one of these devices reaches the level required to produce legislative control or informal sanctions (e.g., in the case of the trampoline), new devices will be developed to produce new thrills—and new morbidity.

This relationship between the routinization of work and the attractiveness of high-risk, active recreation is not a matter of speculative, arm-chair sociology. Research data are beginning to accumulate which show that those individuals who express low levels of job satisfaction and who in fact have low levels of educational and occupational achievement are most likely to engage in high-risk activities, such as sky-diving and snowmobiling, are most likely to prefer the higher horsepower models in outboard engines and in automobiles, and are likely to "live dangerously" not merely in the restricted area of highway behavior but in many areas of their lives (Carlson and Klein, 1970; see also Waller, 1969). The huge increase in the average horsepower of an outboard motor and in the number of such motors in use during the past decade, the explosive growth in popularity of the snowmobile in the past two years (and the explosive increase in death and injury produced by this machine), and the substantial increases in the ownership of high-horsepower automobiles and private aircraft are not attributable to affluence alone. (After all, the affluent individual could have opted for a harpsichord, a tennis racket, or a potter's wheel—devices which involve rather low morbidity and mortality.) At least part of this increase in high-energy, high-risk devices seems clearly attributable to the transfer of the cultural demands from the area of production to the area of consumption.

The Adolescent—a Special Problem

The American adolescent male provides us with a specific illustration of this general process. As a result of the rising standard of living, he is reaching biological maturity at an earlier age than was true two or three decades ago (Seybald, 1968). And as a result of our society's increasing technological sophistication, his access to a meaningful role in the occupational scene occurs several years later than it used to. This means that for a period of five to ten years he remains in a situation in which he has internalized the cultural demands but has little opportunity to express them productively. Since only a few adolescents can achieve distinction through academic success, athletic skills, student government, or other legitimate channels, many of them are virtually forced to seek distinction and status in such recreational areas as hot-rodding, motorcycling, surfing, sky-diving. For many adolescents, knowledge about automobiles, ingenuity in modifying them, and virtuosity in driving them may provide the only route to status among peers and to some sort of equality with adults. Some adolescents indicate, by their driving, that they want to be not equal to but "more equal than" adults—but this is not the main point. To the extent that adolescents are forced to use the automobile to satisfy the cultural demands that they have been taught, they are necessarily increasing their exposure—and this alone will increase the number of crashes, regardless of the quality of their driving. This increase is unlikely to be reversed until the adolescent can be given a more meaningful role in our society.

Here again, this is not speculation. There are increasingly good data to indicate that adolescent males who are least successful in school or in other enterprises appropriate to their age group are most likely to be involved in the traffic violations and to be in conflict with school authorities and the police in connection with deviant behavior that permits them to demonstrate individual initiative and to take risks (Carlson and Klein, 1970; Schuman *et al.*, 1967).

The Role of Violence in
American Society

The singling out of violence as a conspicuous aspect of our culture has by now become a cliché—but the very fact that it is so thoroughly taken for granted has powerful implications for the accident rate.

There is now good evidence that at least for some children exposure to violence on television produces an increase of aggressiveness in their play—an aggressiveness that undoubtedly contributes to their injury rates. The broadcasters have recently agreed to reduce fantasy violence in the Saturday morning television cartoon programs. But the government of the United States has not shown similar social responsibility by eliminating the Vietnam war, the violent aspects of which receive considerable and continuous exposure via television and the other mass media.

The violence from the radical right and the radical left, and that between militants and civil authorities, undoubtedly also influences the accident rate, because, as Waller (1969) has shown, the distinction between unintentional and intentional violence is rather tenuous. And Waller's research data, as well as the over-all statistics on firearms deaths, tend to reinforce the recent prediction that the huge numbers of guns purchased during the past three or four years by whites for protection against black militants are likely to kill far more friends, relatives, and neighbors by accident than black looters and rioters by intention.

Some Implications for Action Programs

If the views set forth in the foregoing pages are valid—that is, if a significant proportion of accidents are the inevitable result of a discrepancy between the cultural demands and the social and technological reality—three courses of action suggest themselves. First, one can attempt to modify the social and technological reality. Secondly, one can attempt to modify the cultural demands. Thirdly, one can attempt to alleviate the consequences of those injuries that will occur inevitably as long as the discrepancy persists.

Modifying the social and technological reality seems the least feasible and the least desirable course. Whatever the merits of a nineteenth-century social and technological order—and they were substantially fewer than some nostalgic romantics by Barry Goldwater out of Norman Rockwell would have us believe—they did not include a standard of living that even remotely approached the one to which, rightly or wrongly, we have become attached. And so, as John Kenneth Galbraith has emphasized, if we want a society which includes mass education, jet travel, the proliferation of labor-saving devices, and two automobiles in every garage, we can have it only at the price of a technology which does *not* permit a substantial number of people to satisfy the current cultural demands in the sphere of production. On the contrary, if present trends continue, more and more of us will have to satisfy more and more of the cultural demands through leisure-time, consumption activities.

Modifying the cultural demands seems somewhat more feasible. Indeed, some evidence has been accumulating over the past two decades to indicate that they are in fact changing—though very slowly. College students—even those who are living in dormitories rather than in hippie communes—are demonstrating greater concern with societal and community welfare and less with individual achievement than their counterparts of twenty years ago. And on an individual level they seem more interested in achieving a humane, cooperative style of life than high personal distinction through aggressive competition. But given the present state of the educational enterprise and the mass media, these changes will be a long time in pervading our society as a whole.

The remaining alternative, therefore, is to alleviate the consequences of those injuries that are inevitable instead of futilely attempting to prevent their occurrence—and this can be accomplished in two ways. First, we can attempt to reduce the amount of injury incurred. If an individual actively seeks risks, the successful incorporation of effective safeguards into a recreational device is likely to send him in search of a less safe device. But even if he seems to be courting hazard, incorporation of damage-reducing features can protect him from the more serious ranges of injury. Thus, every attempt must be made to encourage the development of passive countermeasures such as air bags and energy-absorbing vehicle designs, flameproofing of materials, shatterproofing of glass, and to enforce the use of active countermeasures such as motorcycle helmets. The basic principles and techniques for this approach have been understood for years (Haddon, 1970). It is not a lack of feasibility that impedes their implementation.

Secondly, the quantity and quality of emergency medical care are even more in need of improvement than is the case with general medical care. When we realize that the major cause of death in 20 to 25 percent of highway fatalities is not the initial injuries but inadequate or incompetent emergency care, and when we realize that this percentage translates to 15,000 lives a year, we may conclude that diverting to medical care some of the resources now used in attempting to prevent injuries which seem culturally determined and hence inevitable might be an effective way of reducing death and suffering.

References

Bhise, V. D., and T. H. Rockwell. Two approaches to a non-accident measure for continuous assessment of safety performance. Unpublished paper, Dept. of Industrial Engineering, Ohio State University, 1968.

Carlson, W. L., and D. Klein. Familial vs. institutional socialization of the young traffic offender. *Journal of Safety Research*, 2(1), March, 1970, 13–25.

Haddon, W., D. Klein, and E. A. Suchman. *Accident Research: Methods and Approaches,* Harper and Row, 1964. (Chapters 9 and 10)

Haddon, W. On the escape of tigers. *Technology Review*, May, 1970, 44–53.

Schuman, S. H., D. C. Pelz, N. J. Ehlrich, and M. L. Selzer. Young male drivers. *Journal of the American Medical Association*, June 19, 1967, 1026–1030.

Seybald, H. *Adolescence: a Sociological Analysis,* Appleton-Century-Crofts, 1968, 134–144.

Thompson, J. D., and D. R. Van Houten. *The Behavioral Sciences,* Addison-Wesley, 1970, 69ff.

Waller, J. A. Accidents and Violent Behavior: Are They Related? in D. J. Mulvihill, M. M. Tummin, and L. A. Curtis, *Crimes of Violence, A staff report to the National Commission on the Causes and Prevention of Violence,* 13(33):1525–1558, Washington, D.C., U.S. Government Printing Office, Dec., 1969.

A Philosophy of Safety and of Safety Education

HERMAN H. HORNE

The author suggests that safety should be perceived as a positive value in harmony with other individual and social values. Safety is a means to an end. Thus, use of the phrase "safety from" is negative whereas "safety for" is positive in outlook since safety allows us to be more effective and efficient in our daily living.

This classic article also presents basic concepts about safety, risk, and safety education as well as criticism of fatalism, determinism, pessimism, and the problem of being too safety conscious.

Safety, in the broad sense of the term, is wholeness of life. In the narrow sense of the term, safety is wholeness of physical life, implying the avoidance of accidents. Safety education is the art of cultivating those knowledges, skills, and attitudes that make for safety. The philosophy of safety and of safety education involves the larger social and even cosmic aspects of these topics.

The universe of which we are a part, that is, the cosmos, is characterized, so the astronomers tell us, by law, harmony, symmetry, and rhythm, and order. Nothing happens in the world at large by chance, everything occurs according to law. Safety for man means only that he is catching step with the universe of which he is a part and which explains his being here at all.

Accidents do not just happen. They are caused. Fatalism is an incorrect philosophy of life. Self-determinism is better. Man himself in his choices

Reprinted from Herman H. Horne, "A Philosophy of Safety and of Safety Education," *Safety Education Digest* (New York: The Center for Safety, New York University, 1940), by permission of The Center for Safety. Copyright © 1940 by The Center for Safety.

is a cause, and in a measure man can control external causes and situations.

Just as there is no universal fate compelling us to have accidents, so there is no such thing as luck in having or avoiding accidents. Luck and chance are names for unrecognized causes. Nothing happens without a cause, though the cause may be obscure. Man lives in a world of causation, with which he can cooperate as a cause himself. Through ignorance, carelessness, or wilfulness, man becomes a victim of the very causes with which he might have cooperated.

Pessimism as a philosophy holds that the world is evil and nothing can be done about it. Buddhism as a religion is built on this foundation. The only salvation consists in ceasing to exist. The philosophy of Schopenhauer is similar. Pessimism is not a satisfactory philosophy for safety education, the whole emphasis of which is that the accidental evils of life can be prevented.

Through safety life is preserved at its best. The highest values of life are conserved by safety. The greatest values of all are personal in character. Lesser values are material in character. Safety preserves both the person and the property. It is important to recognize that personal and property values are related, since someone's personal effort has gone into the making of property and property damage affects in various ways the personality of the owner.

Safety means the preservation of health, without which the productive efficiency of man is lessened. Health is basic to all achievement.

There is an ethical aspect of safety. The individual owes it to himself to maintain his capacity at its highest level; he owes it to those dependent on himself to keep himself going as well as he can; and he owes it to all persons to be considerate of their life, limb, and possessions.

An accident is an ugly thing. The victim presents a sorry spectacle. Property damage is an eyesore. There is something ugly in the character of the person negligently or wilfully rendering life hazardous for himself and others. This aesthetic aspect of safety has been neglected. But it is a real aspect and the aesthetic approach to educational problems is particularly effective.

Events have their logic. They come from antecedents, they lead to consequences. Safety is a phase of good logic in events. Peril means bad logic in some poor thinker's behavior. Bad logic and poor thinking when applied, endanger the innocent with the guilty. It is not enough to say, "He got what was coming to him." Maybe he got more than was coming to him, and certainly his family got more than was coming to it. He should realize these things in advance and improve his logic. Poor logic, when it sacrifices safety, has important social and economic consequences; social in that other persons are involved, economic in that one's expenses are increased and one's income may be lessened.

There are certain moral and spiritual aspects of safety which should be kept in mind, though they may not appear as usual parts of the safety movement. This larger safety avoids the perils to the character of man. These perils in character, such as drunkenness, do very directly menace safety. The moral and spiritual health and integrity of man contribute to his sense of the values of life and so help to safeguard his behavior.

It is not a welcome task to point out to those of us who believe so strongly in safety and in safety education that there are certain pitfalls which we have to avoid. One is the danger of overemphasis on our specialty in relation to the remainder of life and other aspects of education. This means the loss of good perspective. After all, safety is but one important aspect of man's well-being.

Another thing to avoid is becoming too safety conscious. The consequence is the danger of having a mass of inhibitions and a welter of fears. We don't want to develop the "sissy" attitude, and we want life bent on accomplishing something worthwhile, not mainly on getting hurt.

After all, life at its best is taking risks for things worthwhile. The good life is adventuring in the creation of values. "Safety first" is an unethical motto. "Better be safe than sorry" is all right, supposing that we are sorry over the proper things. Safety has its rightful place when no greater value is at stake for which a risk should be taken. Policemen, firemen, and soldiers are taking risks constantly in the line of duty.

Aristotle defined courage as the "golden mean" between cowardice and foolhardiness. The man of courage recognizes danger, does not run into it unnecessarily, and acts in behalf of the greatest good. So with all the virtues—they are "golden means."

We should be safe when there is nothing at stake worth risking one's safety for. On Soldier's Field at Harvard University there is a bronze tablet bearing the words of Emerson:

> *Though love repine and reason chafe*
> *There came a voice without reply:*
> *'Tis a man's perdition to be safe*
> *When for the truth he ought to die.*

Man has always obeyed the injunction to "live perilously." But man has usually sought to reduce the perils of survival. Living perilously is a part of the price civilized man pays for his inventions and his mores. Man cannot surrender his inventions, but, to reduce this peril, he can learn how to live with them.

The greatest anachronism of civilization is warfare. At its worst it is destructive of man and his civilization. At its best it is the last desperate means of man's survival and better than the loss of liberty. Every impulse of the safety movement is against war as a mode of settling international issues. And when war comes, the idea of safety operates to minimize its peril in every way possible.

Safety education aims to make the physical survival of the person possible. As such it is a means to all the good ends of life. Its great contribution is in delivering the person so that the other agencies of the good life may make the personality wholesome. Safety education is not an end in itself; it is a means to all good ends. It takes you where you are going so that you arrive; it protects you while you are there; and then it brings you back so you may go again. We believe in safety because we believe in life.

The motives leading to safety are many. We may desire to avoid pain, or inconvenience, or material loss, or giving others trouble, or being thought unskillful. Or we may desire to make and maintain a good record, or to protect life, especially the lives of children. Perhaps the truest of all safety motives is simple respect for personality, one's own and that of others.

To some, life is too monotonous; they seek to make it less so by taking risks in betting, gambling, and the like. To others, life is too hazardous; they seek to make it less so by reducing risks, as in the various forms of insurance. Safety education is like insurance. It reduces the risk of living and the perils of the risks that must be taken. It does not keep us out of the danger zone, but it makes all danger less dangerous. By protecting the person, it makes possible the enrichment of personality. It is the latest child born into the family of Education, and one of its most promising.

A Typology of Accident Proneness

FREDERICK L. MC GUIRE

The concept of accident-proneness has fallen into disrepute because it cannot be demonstrated statistically to be an enduring trait within large groups of people. However, clinical experience supports the conclusion that "accident-prone" individuals do exist. This article attempts to demonstrate that these two sources of data are not necessarily contradictory. If accident proneness is seen as an occasional trait in some individuals and more enduring in others, it is possible to explain both statistical data which argue against the phenomena and clinical observations which support it.

With the introduction of each new implement of force, a certain number of deaths inevitably follow. Many people have been killed because of such devices as the axe, the knife, fire, running horses, gunpowder, airplanes and, of course, the motor vehicle. As I recall, the first recorded automobile accident took place in Ohio around the year 1910, in daylight, in the middle of a broad street, and between the only two cars registered in the state. Since that time Americans have displayed an apparently frantic need to smash and kill themselves on the highway. Even in wartime, the folks at home have usually managed to compile a death rate higher than that incurred by our fighting men overseas, and without the aid of an obliging enemy equipped with modern weapons of war.

It goes almost without saying that many of our highway collisions are influenced by such things as bad vehicle design, poor roads, and traffic

Reprinted from Frederick L. McGuire, "A Typology of Accident Proneness," *Behavioral Research in Highway Safety*, I, No. 1 (1970), by permission of the author and Behavioral Publications, Inc. Copyright © 1970 by Behavioral Publications, Inc., New York.

signs which all too often appear to have been created for the sole purpose of plunging the transportation system into chaos. But it is also apparent that many collisions are the result of inappropriate human behavior. This behavior, while obvious at the time of the accident, sometimes seems so unusual and atypical of the particular individual involved that it is impossible to say that he possesses traits or personal characteristics which distinguish him from accident-free drivers.

Many highway accidents are incurred by people who never before were so involved, have committed few or no violations, have no apparent personality defects, and have no record of illegal or asocial behavior. In fact, most accident-involved drivers seem to fall into this category.

However, there is one group of people who stand apart—the accident prone. For many years we have played with the concept of unequal accident liability or accident proneness, based on the assumption that certain individuals have more than their proportionate share of accidents, further assuming that they were possessed of certain traits or characteristics. It was also hypothesized that these characteristics were stable and enduring over time—perhaps even innate. The concept of so-called accident proneness resulted from the early work of Greenwood, in England (Greenwood, 1919, 1920). He noted and quantified the fact that among female munitions workers during World War I a certain number had more than their share of accidents, that is, the total number of accidents were not evenly distributed. Thus he concluded that some individuals were more likely to incur accidents than others.

This was a fascinating idea, it caught on very quickly, and has persisted practically unchallenged until recent years. In fact, after 1920 Greenwood did not write on the subject again until 1950, nearly 30 years later, thus helping to create a vacuum of scientific activity during which the theory became a catch phrase and gathered momentum (Greenwood, 1950).

The major flaw in the accident-prone concept is the fact that people who have accidents in one period of time are not necessarily those who have accidents in the next. That is, 10 percent of a population may indeed have 90 percent of the accidents during, say, a two-year period, but during the next two years that 10 percent of the population does not include the same individuals. This means that simply because someone has more than his share of accidents than chance would dictate during any one period of time, there is no reason to predict that he will continue to do so. In fact, it has been shown by Forbes, using data gathered by the Bureau of Public Roads in 1938 (more than 30 years ago), that if all accident repeaters during a three-year period were eliminated from the road during the next three years, the accident rate would drop only 4 percent, and that more accident-free drivers would be eliminated than accident producers (Forbes, 1939).

However, the nagging fact remains that some people do have more accidents than others. Repeatedly, we have the experience of seeing people who are obviously engaged in placing themselves in one situation after another in such a way as to increase their chances of having an accident. Furthermore, under our very eyes they amass an impressive array of collisions and injuries. No clinical psychologist or psychiatrist experienced in working with individual patients could ever be convinced by mere theorizing that "accident-prone" people do not exist. The author's files, for example, contain many cases of individuals who have been singularly devoted to the task of systematically flirting with physical disaster—some of them to the point of consciously using the motor vehicle as an instrument of attempted suicide or murder.

Fortunately, these two sources of data are not necessarily contradictory. In fact, together they point to a very likely conclusion, namely, that certain people *are* accident-prone, but sometimes only for short periods of time, and that there are others who are accident-prone over extended periods of time—perhaps for several years or most of their remaining lifetime.

How then, may we put this problem of accident-proneness into perspective? The present discussion offers a proposed typology of the accident-prone individual.

First, however, it must be emphasized that when we are attempting to describe those personal characteristics of individuals which may make them more liable to accidents, we are assuming that risk and exposure are equal. Thus if a person drives 50,000 miles a year and possesses a "low-risk" personality, he may still have a definite accident record; and a person who drives few or no miles per year but possesses many "accident-related" traits may easily have very few accidents. Obviously, high-exposure individuals will tend to have more accidents quite independent of their personal characteristics. In this discussion of what constitutes accident-proneness, it is assumed that exposure and risk are equal.

Type I—Short-Term Accident-Proneness

The primary characteristic of short-term accident-proneness is the fact that the individual is reacting to disruptive influences which originate primarily from external pressures and, once they are relieved, he begins to return to his former state of more favorable adjustment. He may be placed into one of two sub-types.

TYPE IA—CRISIS REACTIONS

This person is placed in a situation or series of situations which is stressful. A man may be in the process of divorcing his wife; his child may be hospitalized by a long-term illness; financial burdens may be pressing in on him; an unmarried woman may be fearful she is pregnant; a college student is worried about low grades, and so on.

Depending upon his basic personality structure and how much help and support is available from others during such times, a person tends to show other symptoms such as forgetfulness, inattention to traffic signals, unusual irritability toward other drivers, and unwillingness to give up the right of way or show routine courtesies, a tendency to speed or throw a car around corners, an unaccustomed use of alcohol, and driving while fatigued due to insomnia.

However, once the crisis is resolved, the person returns to his previous state of good adjustment and he is no longer accident-prone. This period of time may obviously last from several weeks to several months, and occur only once or twice in the lifetime of any particular individual.

However, this is not to say that a Type IA individual is in a minor state of stress. During such periods, people have been known to commit suicide, become alcoholic, and engage in serious asocial and/or anti-social behavior. In some instances the damaging effect of such a life-crisis may persist after the pressures have vanished, and the individual becomes a Type II Accident Repeater.

TYPE IB—REACTIONS TO TRANSIENT CONDITIONS

Many individuals who possess otherwise stable personalities and are not especially threatened by the environment still sometimes find themselves under the influence of pressures which may make them accident-prone. A person may be recovering from an illness which leaves him tired, such as infectious mononucleosis, or he suddenly finds himself working extra hard on the job, which makes him fatigued while driving home on a wintery night in a closed car. In this age of increasing affluence, many people suddenly discover that for some time they have been drinking comparatively heavily, not particularly because of stress or personal need, but in response to the sub-culture in which they find themselves. Such people then may embark on a personal program of curtailed drinking. Many people are given new drugs by a well-meaning physician, only to discover later that in their case, driving ability is impaired, or in combination with other drugs, they no longer are safe drivers.

These conditions which may lead to a period of accident-proneness may be self-terminating or quickly brought under control by the individual once he recognizes what is happening.

Type II—Long-Term Accident-Proneness

The distinguishing characteristic of the Type II individual is that he is under disruptive influences which stem largely from internal sources and, while these pressures may rise and wane, they are relatively constant and always a threat. Type II includes three sub-types.

TYPE IIA—CHARACTER CONDITIONS

A person's character is thought of as comprising those relatively stable traits and behaviors by means of which we tend to characterize him as a person, listing such positive terms as honest, friendly, loyal, courteous, and dependable; or such negative ones as dishonest, mean, rude, and untrustworthy. By and large, character traits are measured against some norm of social conformity, and a person who exhibits asocial or anti-social behavior is often described as having a character disorder.

Individuals in this group are likely to exhibit varying degrees of disrespect for authority and the feelings and rights of others. They may ignore speed limits, run stop signs, engage in drag races or other competitive behavior on the highway, and be generally selfish in their use of the automobile.

By definition, character traits are enduring over time, perhaps for a lifetime. However, a person may change his character as the result of becoming more mature with age, education, the need to be approved of by his employer or other significant persons, marriage, responsibility, threat of retaliation by legal authorities or other social agencies, or simply "slowing down" from old age. Many teen-age drivers would be included in this group. However, labeling them as character disorders for our purpose does not necessarily carry the usual implications of psychopathology, since most of them are reacting "normally" to a particular state of development from which they may be expected to recover.

TYPE IIB—INTRA-PSYCHIC CONDITIONS

These people include those whom we would call neurotic or psychotic—personality deviations in the more traditional clinical sense. Symptoms are extremely varied, including such things as anxiety, depression, inability to concentrate or make decisions, memory disturbances, heightened irritability, morbid doubts, obsessions, irrational fears, insomnia, compulsions, inability to enjoy social relations, tension, fatigue, headaches, gastrointestinal disturbances, and multiple aches and pains. In more serious cases the symptoms may include disorientation, loss of memory, poor speech, suspiciousness, destructiveness, apathy, ideas of reference, and delusions.

Not all neurotic or psychotic persons need be accident-prone, however. For example, the obsessive-compulsive neurotic may be extremely rigid and ultraconforming to traffic rules and regulations. Indeed, an over-concern for safe driving might even be part and parcel of his neurosis. Only those whose symptoms are manifested in such a way as to influence their safe driving are included in this category.

Conditions of this type are usually thought of as being long-term, lasting from several months to many years. However, here too it is possible for persons to change under the influence of time, environmental pressures, and treatment.

TYPE IIC—PHYSICAL CONDITIONS

These are people who are suffering physical conditions which may impair their ability to drive safely, such as failing eyesight, senility, untreated diabetes, seizures not under drug control, and a host of other physical conditions which are likely to persist over a long period of time or become worse.

These types may, of course, overlap or combine to produce accident-proneness in any single individual. For example, a neurotic individual may suddenly be thrust into a life-crisis, a combination of Type IA, crisis reaction, and IIB, intra-psychic condition. A person with definite anti-authoritarian attitudes who makes a practice of defying traffic regulations may incur a physical disability and refuse to either accept it or modify his driving behavior accordingly—a combination of Types IIA and IIC. However, in most cases it should be both possible and useful to distinguish the two or more sources which combine to produce accident-proneness in any one individual.

This view of accident-proneness as something subject to changing classification does not, fortunately, preclude measurement and identification; it merely suggests a change in tactics. Instead of examining a person for traits or characteristics which are relatively enduring over time, such as sex, school, or family history, etc., it becomes necessary to evaluate his life-style as it now exists. For example, while we know that adult individuals with a history of a broken family and school truancy may have a higher accident rate, it becomes necessary to evaluate their present marital state, recent job performance, and the possible existence of any short-term pressures in order to make a more accurate estimate of their accident potential in the immediate future.

By the same token, once we have correctly labeled a person as a safe driver, he must be re-evaluated periodically in order to detect any new possibility that his personal and social environment is changing in the direction of creating accident-producing behavior where none previously existed.

Actually, this approach is far from new. Any experienced and capable personnel director will recognize it as the same "common-sense" approach he has been using for years. When an employee's wife suddenly dies, or his child is ill, it is logical to explore the possibility of removing him from the driver's seat of a cross-continental bus, the throttle of a locomotive, or the use of dangerous machinery. It is also in keeping with what we have known about human behavior for a long time—that people are composed of characteristics and traits which are dynamic and changing as well as those which are relatively stable and durable, and that the environment is capable of interacting with and changing both.

However, by this type of conceptualization and organization, we are able to lay a better foundation for an approach to accident-proneness which some of us have defended for many years, namely, that accident-proneness *does* exist in some people for at least short periods of time, exists in others for relatively long periods of time, and is in both instances predictable if properly measured at the right time.

References

Forbes, T. W. The normal automobile driver as a traffic problem. *J. of Gen. Psychol.* 1939, 20, 471–474.

Greenwood, M. Accident proneness. *Biometrika,* 1950, 37, 24.

————, and H. M. Woods. The incidence of industrial accidents upon individuals with special reference to multiple accidents. *Rep. Indust. Res. Bd.* No. 4, London, 1919.

————, and G. U. Yule. An inquiry into the nature of frequency distributions representative to multiple happenings, with particular reference to the occurrence of multiple attacks of disease or of repeated accidents. *J. Roy. Statis. Soc.* 1920, 83, 255.

What You Don't Know Can Hurt You

A. F. SCHAPLOWSKY

Lack of safety knowledge is cited by the author as a cause of several example accident cases. An educational program which stresses why accidents occur rather than the teaching of safety rules provides a solution to this problem of safety ignorance. When people understand how accidents happen, their behavior will be positively influenced; traditional approaches which rely on scare methods or use of statistics are seldom effective.

When your public health department studies those community problems which are affecting its health and well being, accidental injuries and deaths always appear as a major problem. The health officer determines the relative importance of various community health conditions by comparing the number of premature deaths, cases of disability and the amount of lost productivity which they cause.

Accidents continue to be the leading cause of death for individuals in this country between the ages of 1 and 35 years and the fourth leading cause when all ages are considered. The National Health Survey also tells us that each year 10 million people in this country incur a bed-disabling accidental injury and 1.7 million of these are hospitalized. We are told these disabilities result in the annual loss of over 107 million workdays. You can rapidly calculate that this is equivalent to the absence of over 400,000 men from our work force every day.

Today we are at a time in our country's history when every resource,

Reprinted from A. F. Schaplowsky, "What You Don't Know Can Hurt You," *School and College Safety,* National Safety Congress Transactions (Chicago: National Safety Council, 1961), 17–19, by permission of the National Safety Council. Copyright © 1961 by the National Safety Council.

human or material, is vitally needed and therefore, those measures essential to conserve these resources have a special urgency. We cannot continue to afford human losses among our promising young people nor among men and women of age and experience.

All of you know as well as I that accidents can be prevented by bringing about changes in man's environment and in his behavior. Most of us in this room are more concerned with changes in his behavior. We know that behavior may be changed as a result of an increase in man's knowledge, improvement in his skills or modification of his attitudes. We also know that lack of knowledge affects attitudes and beliefs.

In accident prevention we are faced with some of the same thinking that public health and medicine faced with the communicable diseases not too many years ago. Before the causes for various diseases were known, people blamed sickness upon evil spirits or bad air or some other superstitious belief. It was only after specific causes for these diseases were discovered and understood by the people that these beliefs were largely dispelled. Today since the causes of accidents are not generally known, people blame them on luck or chance. As more specific information about the causes of various kinds of accidents become known and are understood these beliefs will also change.

In traffic many accidents can be traced to genuine lack of knowledge about the rules of the road, mechanics of the motor vehicle or the physical laws which govern the performance of the automobile and capabilities of the driver. Yet today there are 85 million drivers and 180 million pedestrians in this country who must have a complete understanding and acceptance of the rules of the road if we are to reduce the number of injuries involving motor vehicles. Many people are still uninformed or misinformed about the advantages of using safety belts in the family car. Yet the evidence is very substantial that the number of serious injuries and deaths could be markedly reduced if a large portion of the motoring public habitually used this simple device.

Lack of knowledge about the quality of air to be used in the compressed air containers used in scuba diving recently resulted in death for two individuals and serious illness for a number of others. It seems these individuals recharged their containers at a local gasoline service station. Unknown to them the air compressor at the station filled their containers with air containing tiny droplets of oil. After breathing this air they developed a form of pneumonia, called lipoid pneumonia, which was difficult to treat. Since pathogenic organisms had not caused the pneumonia it would not respond to the usual drug therapy.

From the large number of accidental poisoning cases among children which involve aspirin, it can be assumed that many adults do not regard aspirin as a medicine or know that it can be poisonous if ingested in large amounts. There is also general lack of knowledge that many common household articles can be poisonous if ingested.

In rural areas the misuse of liquified petroleum products have resulted in many accidental injuries. Since these products are bottled under pressure, they have been used for such things as inflating flat tires on trucks and farm tractors and to provide air pressures for paint sprayers. The users because of lack of knowledge about the explosive and flammable properties of this material were not aware of the possible hazards involved.

Lack of knowledge about the properties of ultra thin plastic bags during the past several years have resulted in their being used in ways which have caused the suffocation of many children. Many mothers without realizing the danger have used these materials to cover pillows or mattresses in baby beds or have left them within reach of small children.

Lack of knowledge about the side-effects of certain drugs such as tranquilizers and antihistamines has resulted in many accidents. It may be particularly dangerous to drive an automobile after taking some of these medications.

All too many deaths are caused each year because the properties of carbon monoxide are not understood. It is difficult to comprehend the dangers of something which is odorless, colorless, and tasteless.

These examples are just a few of many that could be given to illustrate the point that many accidents can be traced to a lack of knowledge by an individual. How can we do a better job of imparting knowledge?

Perhaps we need to be more dramatic and utilize more imagination and ingenuity in preparing our safety educational messages.

Perhaps we also need to give more consideration to helping people recognize and understand the human factors which underlie many accidents. These factors are generally thought to be of three types: physical factors (poor vision and hearing, disease), emotional factors (hate, fear), and physiological factors (fatigue, drugs, alcohol).

It has also been suggested that a list of premonitory signs could be developed to help people recognize when they are not functioning up to par and, therefore, more likely to have an accident. One individual I know has developed a few such warning signals for himself. For example, when he is working in his woodworking shop, if he makes several errors in judgment or in such things as measuring a piece of wood, he regards this as a signal to change his pattern of work or to discontinue work in which he is more likely to injure himself. He has developed similar personal warning signals which he uses in driving his automobile. He believes helping people to recognize such individual premonitory signs may be more fruitful in reducing accidents than trying to impress upon people all the possible hazards in their environment.

Perhaps we need to concentrate more on teaching people the "why" of safety gadgets or rules rather than insisting that people simply learn the rules, use the gadgets, or adopt a safe behavior. When an individual learns why he does a thing a certain way, his precautions become a part of him. In talking to a group about the advantages of using a safety belt in their automobile, one is likely to succeed in having them recognize the value of the device if they can see a film for example, which shows what happens to occupants with and without seat belts in an automobile when it is involved in a collision. He may not be as successful if he shows them pictures of the gory results of accidents or tries to impress them with the statistical results of the research.

When we help people to understand how accidents happen, we are helping them want to be safe and helping them to recognize that accidents, like diseases, have causes.

As an example of helping people understand the causes of accidents, let me briefly describe a project that the Public Health Service has supported during the last few years. This project was located in Mississippi County, Ark., where the number of fires and burn injuries and deaths were unusually high when compared to other sections of the country.

One man was assigned to the local health department and he developed a program using the traditional public health approach in attacking a new problem. The approach essentially follows these steps: defining the problem, selecting an appropriate solution, and applying the solution.

In defining the problem, an extensive reporting system was set up in order that all information about fires and burns could be assembled and studied. A comprehensive investigation of most of the fires occurring in the county was conducted in order to obtain information about all factors possibly related to causation. As a result of the information gathered, it was learned that most of the fires were caused by inadequate electrical wiring, misuse of petroleum products, and poor installation of heating and cooking stoves.

In relation to these causes, it was also determined that many residents did not know the purpose of the fuse in the electrical system and in general just how the electrical system worked. There was misunderstanding about the properties of gasoline and kerosene. Individuals did not understand that the vapors given off by gasoline are heavier than air and that gasoline was explosive only when its vapors became mixed with air. There was general lack of information about the flammability of other materials like hair sprays and fingernail polish removers.

The solution to the problem seemed to be the development and conduct of an educational program directed at eliminating these deficiencies. Such a program was developed. It was made as simple and yet as dramatic as possible. Intensive efforts were made to reach a large percent of the total population of the county.

Some Techniques for Teaching

A good teacher uses a variety of approaches and adapts his methodology to the needs of students and the unique characteristics of the lesson. In planning and conducting lessons, the teacher is encouraged to refer to this article for help in selecting and applying appropriate learning activities. That people learn best when given the opportunity to become personally involved in learning experiences is a good general principle to follow.

It is hoped that this information will be helpful to the teacher as he involves those whom he instructs. There is great need for better instructors in safety and other fields.

Presented here is a ready reference of some of the techniques and tools for teaching and leading discussion groups. This presentation does not intend to treat all the techniques and tools for teaching. Neither has an attempt been made to discuss each technique fully.

The following teaching techniques are outlined briefly:

Brainstorming	Lecture
Buzz Session	Panel, Symposium
Case Study	Problem Solving
Demonstration	Question-Answer
Discussion	Role Playing
Group Procedure	Special Report
Incident Process	

These outlines are followed by a brief discussion of teaching tools.

I. *Brainstorming*

A. Definition: Brainstorming is a group attempt to solve a well-defined problem by offering any solution which comes to mind, no matter how extreme. This technique attempts to generate ideas quickly and in large quantity by the free association of ideas while suspending all criticisms. It is "using the *brain* to *storm* a problem."

B. Utilization

1. For coming up with different ways of presenting leadership lessons.
2. For planning special projects.
3. For helping to solve specific individual problems.
4. Especially beneficial for the more able people who need help in channeling and directing their thinking.
5. When a group bogs down on a problem, brainstorming may pave the way to a solution.
6. When application of an idea is desired, brainstorming can suggest many applications which no one individual could think of.

C. Procedure

1. Select a problem and state it clearly and specifically.
2. Designate a recorder who will list all ideas on the chalkboard, or newsprint if a chalkboard is not available.
3. Rule out all critical judgments, negative comments, and evaluation.
4. Keep the setting informal and relaxed.
5. Encourage free flow of ideas no matter how far out or freewheeling.
6. Encourage building on to ideas, combining, or improving them.
7. Make suggestions only to keep thinking active, to open up new lines of thought.
8. Close the session after 15 to 20 minutes.
9. Restate the problem and move into the sorting out and refining period.
10. Evaluate the ideas objectively without giving blame or credit.
11. Narrow the ideas to one final solution.
12. Summarize.

13. If possible, contact each participant the following day for afterthoughts which often are of a higher quality than the original ones.

D. Tools: Chalkboard or newsprint sheets.

E. Advantages

1. Everybody participates.
2. With the ground rule that no idea may be criticized, many bright ideas can appear quickly.
3. One idea can spark off other ideas in rapid succession.
4. Brainstorming often frees the individual to be more creative and productive than he usually is.
5. A spirit of fun and congeniality can bring the members close together.

F. Disadvantages

1. Difficult in a large group. Better results may be obtained by breaking up into groups of from eight to fifteen.
2. Unless guided properly, a group may begin criticizing and evaluating before all the ideas are out.
3. Is more effective if the group is made up of people of approximately the same training or rank.
4. Is not a substitute for other types of conference.

II. Buzz Session

A. Definition: A buzz session or group is a short-term device used to divide a large group into sub-groups of three to six persons to consider a specific, limited problem or question for three to eight minutes. The smallness of the sub-group enables each member to participate; the shortness of the time requires each to work hard and on target.

B. Utilization

1. To warm up a large group for general discussion.
2. To overcome a feeling of helplessness or apathy and to direct a group toward action.
3. To obtain a cross section of ideas, opinions, suggestions, decisions in a minimum of time with maximum participation.

4. To give everyone a chance to contribute.
5. To take time out for quick assessment of additional data, materials, suggestions.
6. To set up an agenda for a meaningful learning experience in the total group.
7. To test a set of ideas and to increase communication between the speaker and the audience.

C. Procedure

1. Give a survey presentation of the problem to the large group.
2. Subdivide the group into sub-groups—buzz groups of three to six persons, each group to meet by itself. Count off one to three or one to six, or use any other quick method.
3. Specify and limit the problem for buzz group discussion. Write it large on a chalkboard or newsprint for everyone to see and to understand clearly. Every buzz group may work on the same problem, or each group may be given a facet of the problem.
4. Quickly, appoint a chairman and a recorder in each buzz group.
5. Director circulates among the groups to keep them on target.
6. Each buzz group prepares a concise written or oral report of its recommendations, decisions, or whatever action was called for.
7. Reconvene for sub-group reports. If every group had the same problem, call for one item from each group in turn, so that the first group does not give all the points at once.
8. Director summarizes the findings.

D. Tools: Paper and pencil, chalkboard, newsprint, or acetate sheets where reports are to be projected on the screen with the overhead projector.

E. Advantages

1. Small size of buzz group permits everyone to participate and to express himself, resulting in a variety of ideas and opinions in a short time.
2. Small groups work better and faster because they know that they have no time to waste and will have to come up with a group report.

3. Easier and faster to obtain better choices and agreements from each of the six groups of five persons apiece than from a total group of thirty people.
4. Group feelings throughout the main group can be readily obtained.
5. Each sub-group must take responsibility for its own operation and for its expressions.
6. Pride is established and morale is boosted in everyone in himself and in his sub-group by his individual contribution.
7. Surprisingly less time is required to obtain fuller agreement or a better solution in the reconvened large group.
8. Little equipment needed beyond paper and pencil and chalkboard.

F. Disadvantages

1. If the director fails to choose the right moment to initiate buzzing, the sub-groups might find little purpose of interest in buzzing.
2. If the problem for buzzing is not clearly defined, limited, and understood, the sub-group members might become frustrated and the buzz results will be poor.
3. Not providing a time limit might allow the participants to just visit or to over-develop their decisions.

III. Case Study

A. Definition: A case study is an analysis and a solving of a problem that might be typical. It is an open-end proposition with "What would you do?" The solution must be practical and the best under the circumstances.

B. Utilization

1. Especially useful for analyzing personal problems of people.
2. Good method for training people to participate orally (under the close attention of others), to think through, to feel vicariously the roles of the persons concerned in the problem.
3. Excellent for teaching persons to be open to suggestions, viewpoints, and feelings of others.
4. Trains one how to deal with himself and with others before facing the real thing.

C. Procedure: The case method is essentially a problem-solving technique which leads thinking through effective group discussion supplemented with role playing.

   1. A group of four or five persons is headed by a trained leader, who oversees but does not dominate the study.

   2. The members seek individual solutions of the problem by critical examination of the data and through frank discussion in the group.

   3. A summary of observations, opinions, and preliminary conclusions is made on a chalkboard.

   4. Each person then writes out what action he would take, if confronted with that or a similar problem, and defends his decision before the group.

   5. Finally, the entire group formulates one solution, and, if the case had a previous solution, a comparison is made and differences are noted and discussed, and the group's answer is modified, if necessary.

   6. Each participant should leave the study with a clear understanding as to how he would handle a similar problem if he met it in reality.

D. Tools: The nature of the particular problem, its circumstances, the available information, and other factors will decide what tools or aids are useful in the study. Experts, witnesses, and subjects may be called. Among audio-visual aids, useful ones frequently include paper, chalkboards, charts, diagrams, films, pictures, tables of data, tests, objects, models, samples, and tapes, and appropriate equipment associated with aids.

E. Advantages

   1. The case approach is the best substitute for reality: the investigator must analyze and solve selected case problems from real life, but without suffering the problems and the consequences of failure. By putting himself into the roles of the examiner and of the examined, he becomes sensitive to the many factors that may enter a problem.

   2. The smallness of the group (about five or six persons) permits and requires each member to participate fully, and to think through what he might do, if the problem were his. Each one must open up, overcome shyness, speak up, learn to give and take, respect the thinking of others, and be unbiased in his viewpoint and judgment.

3. The deliberations require that one be clear and specific in introducing a problem, be concise in assembling appropriate data, and be logical, reasonable, and practical in summarizing and in formulating a workable solution.
4. The solution of the case is the concentrated effort of several alert minds, and so should be better than that of one mind.

F. Disadvantages

1. Insufficient and inadequate information and being in too much of a hurry can lead to inappropriate results.
2. If the leader fails to arouse the participants to a free flow of ideas, discussions, and decisions, the method may fail to develop the participants appropriately and to obtain a good solution.

IV. Demonstration

A. Definition: A demonstration is a visual presentation of one or more techniques, processes, skills, facts, concepts, or principles to be learned. Someone, often assisted by others, goes through the motions or processes of showing, doing, illustrating and explaining. (It is one of the most effective methods of teaching.)

B. Utilization

1. Certain mental processes involved in developing concepts are best explained by examples—through showing.
2. Is a means of helping people achieve their goals.
3. Can involve one or many of the group members, depending on the demonstration.

C. Procedure

1. Re-examine the objective of the lesson or discussion before giving the demonstration.
2. Practice the demonstration. Never give one without a trial run, because there is always the possibility that it may not work.
3. Make sure that all needed equipment and materials are on hand before starting the demonstration.
4. Seat people so everyone can see and hear.
5. Explain the purpose and prepare the people in advance what to look for.

6. Keep the directions simple; vary the tempo to suit the group.

7. Check periodically during the demonstration to know that each step is being followed.

8. Whenever possible, involve the people in the demonstration.

9. Use vocabulary understood by all.

10. Don't prolong the demonstration. It should usually not exceed twenty-five minutes.

11. Summarize and briefly review, with the group, the key points of the demonstration after it has been concluded.

D. Tools: Chalkboard, tapes, slides, filmstrips, pictures, posters, graphs, maps, charts, and other aids as the demonstration requires.

E. Advantages

1. Is basically concrete instead of being abstract.

2. Showing often involves the learner's first-hand contact with what is referred to in a concept; the impact is extremely vivid.

3. Can clarify points during a lesson.

4. Can heighten interest and increase learning.

5. Good experience for the demonstrators.

6. Showing and telling are better than mere showing or telling.

7. Provides a break from the repetition of lectures.

F. Disadvantages

1. Requires careful planning and rehearsal and can be time consuming.

2. Requires assembling of equipment, supplies, and materials, and sometimes getting extra help.

3. Usually involves only a few people, frequently only the demonstrator.

4. If the group is too large, those in the rear may not be able to see and hear everything.

5. The attention span of the viewers varies in proportion to how meaningful the demonstration is.

V. *Discussion*

A. Definition: Discussion is a group activity in which the leader and the group members cooperatively talk over some problem or topic. It is a process of thinking aloud together.

B. Utilization

 1. Useful for teaching.
 2. For working over concepts which have already been presented to the group, in order to make them clear.
 3. In analyzing problems of common concern to the group.
 4. Valuable for both motivating the participants and enabling them to comprehend the meaning of what they are learning.
 5. In terms of learning, the concept that is discussed, however haltingly, is usually more lasting than the unvoiced concept.
 6. Can be used to improve the speaking and listening skills of the participants.

C. Procedure

Major responsibilities of the group discussion leader are to:

 1. Start the discussion.
    a. Discussion goals must be clearly defined and be understood by the participants.
    b. A circular seating arrangement will help increase interest and participation.
 2. Keep the discussion on the topic. Sometimes the leader may ask a recorder to summarize for the group.
 3. Recognize and involve, if possible, all individuals within the group. Stimulate thinking by asking thought questions; at the same time, encourage each person to do his own thinking.
 4. Devote time to periodic summaries.
    a. Leader would take time to ask, "Where are we?" "What have we been doing?" "Do we have an answer?"
    b. Encourage the participants to evaluate the progress of their discussion.

Some ways of starting discussions:

 1. Introducing challenging topics.
 2. After viewing motion pictures, bulletin board displays, or objects brought to a meeting.
 3. After listening to a tape recording or record.

D. Advantages

 1. Allows everyone to participate.
 2. Provides for the informal expression of personal experiences and information not included in formal written materials.
 3. Permits both leader and member leadership.

4. In thinking aloud together, individual errors in judgment can be revised.
5. When ideas are carefully explored and considered, the finished product represents the thinking of many individuals.
6. Makes participants take sides, defend their points of view, and then live with the consequences.
7. Learner becomes an active participant in the learning process.
8. Involves creative thinking.
9. Helps to develop respect for others even though rejecting their points of view.

E. Disadvantages

1. Is not as effective with large groups as with small, because many will not have a chance to participate orally.
2. Unless the leader encourages a maximum of participation by the members, a few talkative members may end up monopolizing the time.
3. Discussion has to be on a topic or issue that is common knowledge to the participants, because a fruitful discussion can only proceed from the known.
4. It is time consuming.
5. Sometimes the leader cannot tell exactly how much or what the participants have learned.
6. Without good leadership, the discussion may get off the track.

VI. Incident Process

A. Definition: The incident process is a method of learning how to solve problems and work out decisions by studying actual incidents that involve real people in real situations. (This is a less formal, less demanding form of case study.)

B. Utilization—Useful in giving practice in analyzing particular problems.

C. Procedure

1. A written statement of an incident is made. It does not provide all necessary facts for making a decision. The group

is required to take the role of a responsible person and make a decision.

2. Members try to recreate the action by asking the instructor questions concerning relevant facts and clues. They try to learn what happened, to whom, when, where, and how.
3. A group member summarizes the facts at the end of this phase.
4. Each member makes and submits his own decision for action in the incident.
5. The group evaluates actions, decisions, and consequences.
6. The group discusses what was useful, what caused difficulties and how they could have been avoided.
7. The group generalizes on how to do better by using some of the effective methods, avoiding action which brings difficulty.

D. Advantages

1. There is a common goal if the group is made up of members from one organization.
2. Easy to share understanding and pool experience.
3. Helps members to think clearly, to appreciate feelings, and to improve in practical judgment.

E. Disadvantages

1. Good case reports require considerable study before discussion, and some members will not have time to prepare adequately.
2. Incomplete case reports lead to guesswork.
3. Group discussion can become limited to members who are adequately prepared.
4. Case discussion may lead to argument rather than discussion.

VII. Group Procedure

A. Definition: Group procedure is a method of having several persons working together on a task that requires their cooperation. (Involvement of people in group procedures highlights the old proverb "hear and forget, see and remember, *do and understand*.")

B. Utilization

 1. Use group discussion method as a means of identifying, analyzing, and solving problems.
 2. When a big job has to be done in a short time, it can be divided into smaller parts and given to small groups (committees).
 3. When there are many jobs to be done, each job can be done by a separate group.
 4. Planning for an occasional event may be done by a small group.
 5. When a group has varied interests, those with similar interests can work together.
 6. Group work, with its considerable stress on initiative and independence, gives people a chance to improve in these areas.
 7. Use different procedures for different purposes. Some procedures are whole-group discussions, small study groups, buzz groups, panel or round table, symposium, debate, role playing, and case studies.

C. Procedure

 1. Select group procedures that will best help the members reach specified goals.
 2. For member-directed group activities, make sure the members understand the purpose of the activity and exactly how it is to be accomplished.
 3. Assign responsibilities to the participants to insure effective group work.

D. Advantages

 1. Groups do not err as readily as does the average individual.
 2. Groups have a larger percentage of correct answers—two heads are better than one.
 3. Group decisions have a stronger effect upon behavior than other learning situations do.
 4. More viewpoints, varied experiences, and wider store of knowledge can be brought to bear on the task.
 5. Discussion encourages mental activities—exchange of ideas can be stimulating and motivational.
 6. Helps individual to give-and-take and to examine all facets of an issue before making a decision.

7. Enables individuals to acquire knowledge that they might not have enjoyed without group effort.
8. Improves the individual's power of self-expression and helps him to take a more active role in subsequent group work. It encourages the development of leadership qualities.
9. Group activities tend to encourage teamwork.

E. Disadvantages

1. Doing things by group methods takes considerable time and effort, especially in the beginning.
2. Discussion in the absence of relevant information is meaningless.
3. The range of the leader's experience determines, in part, how meaningfully he can direct group work.
4. Some leaders are not able to break away from the habit of "telling others what to do."
5. Method can become unwieldy in groups of over fifty people. It is most efficient in groups of twenty-five or less.

VIII. Lecture

A. Definition: The lecture is a formal talk on a specific subject for instruction or information. It is a method of "telling." It is usually a one-way channel of communication.

B. Utilization

1. In presenting the material to large groups in a limited period of time.
2. In introducing new material or an overview of a lesson.
3. In elaborating on the subject.
4. In explaining a process.
5. In bridging gaps between topics to be studied in depth.
6. In explaining difficult points.
7. In summarizing.
8. In reinforcing the written word with oral methods.
9. In providing a change of pace from other methods.

C. Some Ways that May Be Used to Improve the Lecture Method

1. Introduce appropriate visual aids to put the sense of sight to work.

2. Motivate the group by relating the lecture to problems the listeners are familiar with.
3. Express ideas so as to stimulate thinking.
4. Use language which the audience can follow with understanding and interest.
5. Emphasize important points.
6. Return several times to the main thought so that it is emphasized and kept uppermost in mind by the listeners.
7. Get to the conclusion as rapidly as the audience is able to follow.
8. Be sure the ladder of ideas on which the conclusion must stand is clear to the audience.
9. Distribute instruction material, both written and graphic, to supplement the lecture.
10. Open the subject for questions and discussion.
11. Do not read the material word by word.
12. Direct instruction to individuals.
13. Tell the listeners what is expected of them.
14. Develop effective speech habits.

D. Tools

1. Use chalkboard to list the main points of the talk, for outlines, unfamiliar terms, diagrams, and graphs.
2. Use pictures, posters, objects, models, specimens, and flipcharts to illustrate the talk.
3. Use stories, examples, and comparisons to bring out points.
4. Use slides, tapes, and films to clarify meanings.

E. Advantages

1. Saves time.
2. Can cover a lot of material.
3. Can be fully prepared ahead of time.
4. Information that is difficult for the listeners to obtain can be given by the speaker.
5. Present material in an orderly, logical fashion so that it can be clearly understood by the listeners.

F. Disadvantages

1. Puts the learner in the passive role of merely listening.
2. Is often a waste of time, because, being passive, the listeners learn little. (We generally remember only about ten percent of what we hear.)

3. Does not guarantee that the listener will understand its contents.
4. Unless well prepared and delivered, a lecture can become boring to the audience.

IX. *Panel, Symposium*

A. Definition: Panels and symposia are discussion procedures which may be used in either large or small groups. The purpose is to provide an opportunity for a few well-prepared people to discuss a topic of general concern and interest in front of the assembly. (The ideal number of participants is four or five, plus the moderator.) Both procedures are followed by questions or discussion from the floor.

1. Panel: Participants engage in an informal, free exchange of ideas among themselves concerning the topic. The presentations are considered impromptu, but the participants should be well informed.
2. Symposium: Participants, usually with divergent viewpoints, prepare and formally present a set speech (statement) of facts or opinions regarding various facets of the topic. They may then engage in an informal discussion among themselves.

B. Utilization

1. To study a topic in more depth than can be done in a general discussion.
2. Where it is desirable for the members to look for needed information, instead of the leader spoonfeeding the answers.
3. For introduction of new materials; enrichment of the topic being studied; culmination of the study.
4. For motivation.
5. To provide variety in the group procedures.
6. To utilize resource people effectively.

C. Procedure

1. Select a pertinent problem cooperatively with the group.
2. Choose panel or symposium participants carefully, especially the moderator, because the presentation will be no better than those who engage directly in it.
3. All group members may be assigned to prepare for a panel, and then the panelists can be selected extemporaneously.

4. Assist the participants in obtaining the information needed for worthwhile discussion.
5. Have a few practice sessions, if possible.
6. Provide the audience with guidelines on what values and learning to look for during the panel or symposium.

Since much of the success of the presentation depends on the the moderator, his major responsibilities are listed below:

1. Become well versed on the topic.
2. Inform the audience of the topic to be discussed, giving enough background information so that their interest and attention may be aroused and secured.
3. Introduce the members of the panel or symposium.
4. Get the discussion under way, usually by stating a provocative question and then calling upon one of the participants.
5. Guide the discussion—keep the remarks focused on the problem, energize a lagging discussion, bring each participant into the discussion, see that no one monopolizes, make both periodic and final summaries.
6. Stimulate questions and discussion from the audience.

D. Advantages

1. Both the panel and symposium actively involve a number of individuals.
2. Provide opportunity to participants to work together as a group.
3. A given topic can be discussed in depth by a panel or a symposium, whereas it would be difficult in a large group.
4. Can be used to launch small-group discussions in a large group.
5. Change of pace from the usual activities can be refreshing.

E. Disadvantages

1. Only a small number of individuals is directly involved.
2. Even during the question or discussion period, not everyone in the audience can participate.
3. Unless all group members have been given the assignment to prepare for the panel, only the panelists have the benefit of studying the topic in depth.

4. When the participants are well qualified, the procedure is more effective and rewarding.

X. Problem Solving

A. Definition: Problem solving is a method of analyzing problems systematically in order to arrive at solutions. (It is a method richly productive of the highest quality of learning.)

B. Utilization

1. In working on projects.
2. Basically is a means of approaching problems with a searching mind.

C. Procedure

1. Identify the problem, issue, or question requiring an answer or solution, and *define* it specifically so that the members know exactly what they are to do.
2. *Gather evidence* or data that will help in the solution of the problem.
3. Organize and *analyze* the information.
4. *Form a tentative solution* to the problem (hypothesis).
5. *Try out the solution.*
6. If successful, the problem is solved; if not, repeat steps 3, 4, and 5.

D. Advantages

1. Can lead to a good understanding of a problem because it provides for the participants' becoming really involved in their learning.
2. Places emphasis on the members' actively acquiring information and critically examining it, rather than on the leader's presentation of it.
3. Involves not only learning but actual use of what has been learned.
4. Leads individuals through a series of experiences and helps them "discover" basic generalizations themselves—to learn things for themselves, by use of their own abilities.
5. Provides people a chance to learn from their successes and failures.

6. Problem-solving approach to knowledge may be engaged in by all, in varying degrees.
7. Can be used by individuals as well as by groups.

E. Disadvantages

1. Without guidance, individuals may select problems whose solution requires materials and equipment beyond the available resources, or problems too big and unyielding in the time allotted.
2. Unless a problem is defined clearly and sharply, the individuals may flounder in the problem-solving steps and not arrive at a reasonable solution.

XI. *Question-Answer*

A. Definition: The question-answer method is a device wherein the instructor asks questions and the group members reply concerning (a) the retention or remembering of materials presented in lectures, discussions, and assignments; and (b) the stimulation of thinking about concepts, issues, ideas, meanings, and activities of significance, whether or not covered in lectures or assignments.

B. Utilization

1. Good method, if properly used, for stimulating reviews, sparking discussions, arousing interest, opinions, and definitions, and developing deeper thinking.
2. Good springboard for further assignments, particularly away from the book, in response to questions by the members during the period.
3. Should aim at fitting fragments of information into meaningful wholes. A sequence of questions should lead progressively to specific understandings.

C. Procedure

1. Use thought-provoking questions frequently.
2. Use related questions that become progressively more difficult to help participants to acquire concepts in depth.
3. If a question should be answered in a certain way (define, compare, classify, evaluate, etc.), indicate this clearly.
4. Ask questions that are within the range of experience and knowledge of the participants.

5. As a general rule, use some portion of a respondent's answer, if only to encourage him and keep him interested.
6. Include as many members as possible in the questioning. Direct questions to the entire group.
7. It is often better to ask the question and then to call on the individual.
8. Questions may be presented orally, written on the chalkboard, charts, given on typed slips or sheets, flashed on a screen with the opaque or overhead projector, or be taped.
9. An essential part of the question-answer technique involves encouraging members to ask questions.
10. Don't bluff when not sure of an answer. Say "I don't know" and then find out the answer.

D. Tools: Chalkboard, charts, slides, tapes, typed sheets, questions on transparencies for overhead projection.

E. Advantages

1. Convenient device to review the lesson to uncover the known through member responses.
2. Provides checks on whether or not the members did their work, on the instructor's presentation, and on the members' understanding of the lesson or topic.
3. Good personal training in oral expression, in speaking up before a group, and in thinking on one's feet extemporaneously.
4. Wisely selected and carefully phrased questions can contribute substantially to improve learning by stimulating reasoning, evaluating, and generalizing.
5. Gets someone besides the instructor to speak up.

F. Disadvantages

1. Questioning is not profitable when the members don't have a background that will enable them to react intelligently.
2. Questions might be chiefly those which can be answered by "yes" or "no" or by repeating memorized statements from the book.
3. Ambiguous, wordy, or unclear questions can block effective communication.
4. Some instructors tend to specialize in one particular type of question to the exclusion of others.
5. The quality of questioning is limited by the instructor's knowledge of content and his quality of thinking.

6. The instructor might use questioning to substitute for his lack of preparation of the lesson for the day.
7. The instructor's lack of tact might embarrass a person and cause him to withdraw from further participation or involvement.

XII. Role Playing

A. Definition: Role playing is unrehearsed, informal dramatization in which people spontaneously act out human relations problems to become aware of the feelings of someone else, to see a situation through other people's eyes, or to experience how they would act or react in a given situation.

B. Utilization

1. To train in leadership and human relations skill.
2. To train in solving group problems—actual problems can be reenacted.
3. Role playing the characters in a story or situation to make their feelings more real to the group.
4. To figure out how to handle a difficult situation.
5. To teach certain subject content more effectively, such as historical incidents.
6. To give people a chance to say, in a role, what they actually feel rather than what they think you want to hear—they can explore their own feelings and gain insight.
7. Helpful in deepening or changing attitudes, particularly toward members of another ethnic group.

C. Procedure

1. Describe the situation to be role played. "Warm up" the group.
2. Select the role players and ask each one to put himself into the frame of mind of the person he is representing. Emphasize that he is playing a role, not himself.
3. Assign tasks to the audience. Some can put themselves into the shoes of particular actors, or watch for specific events, or judge how realistic the role playing is.
4. Set the stage and start the action. Stop it as soon as it illustrates the problem.
5. Discuss what took place and try to identify the values and

feelings of those involved, and the conditions which caused them to feel or to act as they did.

6. Evaluate and summarize the points learned.
7. Role play may be repeated with the same players reversing their roles or with new players.

D. Advantages

1. Gives people a chance to examine and experiment with roles in situations where actual problems can be worked on. Some mistakes will be made.
2. Enables a person to become aware of and impressed with the thoughts, attitudes, and perspective of someone else, and thus to appreciate the other person's point of view.
3. Participants and observers can put themselves into other people's shoes to experiment with new ways of behaving and to learn by doing.
4. Situations can be devised to fit the needs and interests of the group.

E. Disadvantages

1. Unless the group is sensitive and open-minded enough to try new ways of working together, the role playing may be superficial and fail to produce desired results.
2. Players often tend to "ham up" their parts and make the role play mere entertainment.
3. The director must plan it carefully to keep it at the level of understanding and maturity of the group.
4. Can backfire if suddenly thrust upon the uninitiated.
5. Can be time consuming, depending on the situations enacted.

XIII. Special Report

A. Definition: A special report is a means of getting some particular information before the group, in cases where the data are not generally available to the group but are essential to the lesson or discussion.

B. Utilization

1. To report an interview with an important person.
2. To show research findings which will strengthen the lesson or discussion.

3. To bring in data, whether from books or specialist, which are needed to make the lesson more meaningful.
4. To report on a committee meeting or conference which has bearing on the lesson.

C. Procedure

1. Assignments should be planned well ahead, and the persons making the reports should have enough time to research the topics properly.
2. Content and extent of the assignment should be made clear, suggestions made as to where to find the material, and examples of similar reports made available, if possible.
3. Report, when given, should not be read word for word. The person reporting should be assisted to make his presentation interesting through careful planning and utilization of appropriate teaching aids.
4. Copies of the report may be given to the group members, so that they may follow it during the report or study it beforehand if it is distributed earlier.
5. Presentation should use only part of the lesson or discussion period, so that questions, comments, and discussion may be permitted.
6. Oral reports can become monotonous if the group has to listen to several, one following the other. Space reports between other activities.

D. Tools: In addition to a written report or the outline of the reports, the following tools are often useful in presenting the material effectively: chalkboard, charts, diagrams, maps, pictures, sketches, tables, graphs, posters, models, love items, tapes, assisted by needed projectors and recorders, and even resource people.

E. Advantages

1. Extends the lesson content beyond the instructor, the text, and the classroom into the library and to other resource points.
2. The research, preparation, and presentation develop the individuals doing the assignment.
3. Acquaints those reporting with expanded sources for information and teaches logical organization.
4. Provides more experience in preparing written reports and delivering oral reports to group members.
5. Relieves the instructor of much additional work.

F. Disadvantages

    1. If the assignments, reports, and presentations are not planned well, they can miss the point, wander around, be boring, and be quite wasteful of time and effort.

    2. Assignment directly involves only a few individuals.

    3. Unless the report is presented interestingly, it will not gain the attention of the group.

XIV. Teaching Tools

Teaching tools or audio-visual materials are powerful aids in teaching when used properly; they are not a substitute for real teaching. They enable the instructor or discussion leader to clarify points and encourage more participation by the group. Because they have eye, ear, and often touch appeal, they can make learning interesting and vivid.

A. *Some types of teaching tools:*

Materials

Pictures	Filmstrips
Posters	Globes
Charts	Models
Flipcards	Mockups
Newspapers	Objects
Graphs	Specimens
Maps	Realia
Diagrams	Tape Recordings
Slides	Phonograph Recordings

Equipment

Movie Projector	Radio
Overhead Projector	Television
Opaque Projector	Chalkboard
Slide Projector	Bulletin Board
Filmstrip Projector	Flannel Board
Tape Recorder	Slip Board
Record Player	Magnetic Board

B. *How Teaching Tools Can Help Learning*

    1. Reduce talk. Can help make ideas and concepts clear; make words and phrases real.

2. Increase permanence of learning. A person remembers longer what he sees than what he merely hears.
3. Add interest or motivation.
4. Stimulate involvement and self-activity. The learner may get insights which may encourage him to learn more on his own.
5. Provide for more uniform understanding of what is being studied. Everyone sees the same things.
6. Help meet differences in individual needs, abilities, and experiences.
7. Furnish understanding of involved processes.
8. Afford experiences not easily obtainable through other means.

C. Some general *principles* concerning the use of audio-visual materials:

1. Select teaching aids carefully. Consider suitability, level of understanding, visibility, clearness, ease of presentation, availability of material.
2. Use various aids. No one type of material should be used to the exclusion of others.
3. Prepare materials carefully. Audio-visual aids cannot teach by themselves.
4. Check out all equipment before using it with the group. Try out everything under conditions similar to those when the group meets.
5. Guide the group members through the activity.
   a. Point out what to look for and what to listen for. To explain what the group is seeing or hearing, a study guide is often helpful.
   b. Follow up the activity to clear any misunderstandings and to bridge any gaps in the presentation.

D. Some *abuses* in the use of audio-visual materials:

1. Poor selection of materials.
2. No relation to subject under consideration.
3. Lack of adequate preparation before using.
4. Inadequate follow-up or none at all.
5. Use of too many materials.
6. Use of only one type of material.
7. Use of materials merely to fill up time.
8. Use of materials in rooms not suitable for the purpose.

XV. Using Different Kinds of Aids

A. *Chalkboard:* Because the chalkboard is used extensively, the following are some hints for proper usage:

1. Keep it clean.
2. Write with bold, strong lines.
3. Use legible penmanship.
4. Make the letters and drawings large enough and high enough on the board to be seen.
5. Check for visibility from all parts of the room from time to time.
6. Do not cover up the material on the board by standing in front of it.
7. Use colored chalk for added interest and to differentiate between parts.
8. Do not put too much material on the board at one time unless the specific purpose makes this necessary.
9. Use stick figures or cartoon techniques for dramatizing and adding sparkle to chalkboard teaching.
10. If a drawing is complex, put it on the board before the group assembles.
11. Use the opaque projector in transferring to the chalkboard useful but hard-to-draw diagrams, figures, pictures, charts, etc.
12. Do not put unnecessary and time-consuming accuracy into a drawing when accuracy is not called for.
13. Forms that are regularly used can be painted on the board. Occasionally a dramatic visual presentation can be made by preparing materials on the board in advance and covering it with strips of paper which will be removed, one by one, as the demonstration proceeds.
14. Use templates for diagrams, outlines, etc., which have to be drawn repeatedly.
15. Keep the board looking neat and orderly.

B. *Pictures, posters, charts, diagrams, graphs, maps, objects, specimens, etc.*

1. Select only those which will illustrate the lesson.
2. Make sure that they are large enough to be seen by the entire group.
3. To lessen distraction, cover material prepared for use or display later in the lesson.

4. Uncover one section of a chart or display as it is needed.
5. Point out the main features or characteristics which should be noticed.
6. Display material long enough for everyone to absorb the message.
7. Mount flat items on a firm background for suitable display.
8. Avoid passing items around the room because this results in divided attention.

C. *Projectors*

1. Try them out beforehand.
2. Have them set up and ready to go.
3. Have on hand extra exciter, projection, and other lamps, as necessary.
4. Use stable projector stand, not stacks of books.
5. Tie cords to the leg of the projection stand. Place them so that people will not trip over them.
6. Have materials to be projected in proper sequence for showing.
7. Make sure that everyone can see all of the projected image on the screen.
8. Keep the path clear for the light from the projector to the screen.
9. Darken room sufficiently for good viewing.
10. Focus properly.
11. Do not use lettering or figures that are too small to be read easily when projecting with the overhead, opaque, or slide projectors.
12. Speak loudly enough to be heard over the projector noise.

index

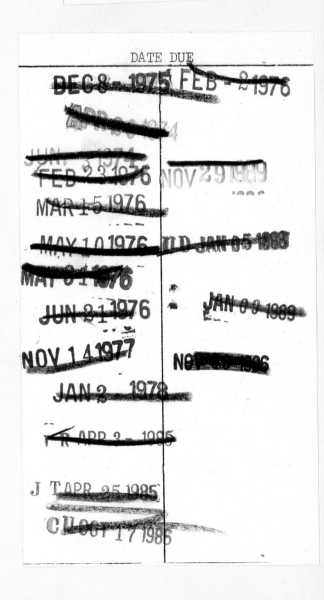

DATE DUE

DEC 8 - 1975   FEB - 2 1976

APR 30 1974

JUN 3 1974
FEB 23 1976   NOV 29 1989

MAR 15 1976

MAY 10 1976   JAN 05 1988

MAY 9 1976

JUN 21 1976   JAN 09 1989

NOV 14 1977   NO   86

JAN 2 1978

R APR 2 1995

J T APR 25 1985

OCT 17 1986